Fundamentals of Amputation Care and Prosthetics

Fundamentals of Amputation Care and Prosthetics

Editor

Douglas Murphy, MD
Associate Professor of Physical Medicine and Rehabilitation
Virginia Commonwealth University
Staff Physician
Hunter Holmes McGuire VA Medical Center
Richmond, Virginia

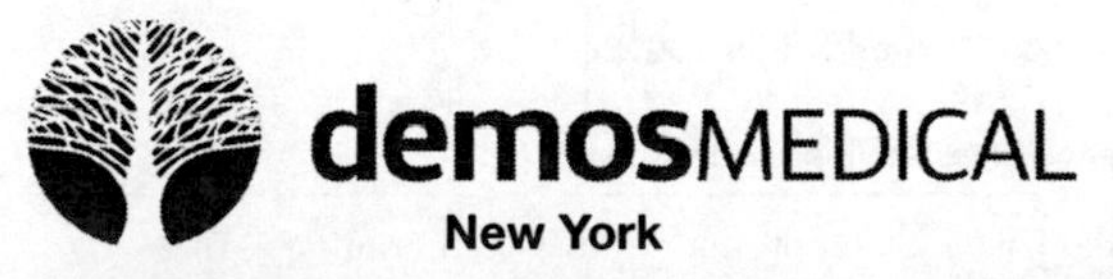

Visit our website at www.demosmedpub.com

ISBN: 9781936287703
e-book ISBN: 9781617051197

Acquisitions Editor: Beth Barry
Compositor: Exeter Premedia Services Private Ltd.

Medicine is an ever-changing science. Research and clinical experience are continually expanding our knowledge, in particular our understanding of proper treatment and drug therapy. The authors, editors, and publisher have made every effort to ensure that all information in this book is in accordance with the state of knowledge at the time of production of the book. Nevertheless, the authors, editors, and publisher are not responsible for errors or omissions or for any consequences from application of the information in this book and make no warranty, expressed or implied, with respect to the contents of the publication. Every reader should examine carefully the package inserts accompanying each drug and should carefully check whether the dosage schedules mentioned therein or the contraindications stated by the manufacturer differ from the statements made in this book. Such examination is particularly important with drugs that are either rarely used or have been newly released on the market.

Library of Congress Cataloging-in-Publication Data
Fundamentals of amputation care and prosthetics / [edited by] Douglas Murphy.
p. ; cm.
Includes bibliographical references and index.
ISBN 978-1-936287-70-3—ISBN 978-1-61705-119-7 (e-book)
I. Murphy, Douglas (Douglas P.), editor of compilation.
[DNLM: 1. Amputation. 2. Artificial Limbs. WE 170]
RD553
617.5'8059—dc23

2013020149

Printed in the United States of America by Gasch Printing.
13 14 15 16 17 / 5 4 3 2 1

Dedicated to David X. Cifu, MD
and the Amputation System of Care
for their exemplary and selfless service to veterans
across the nation.

Contents

Contributors

Christopher Fantini, MSPT, CP, BOCO Lead Clinical/Research Prosthetist, Department of Veterans Affairs, Prosthetics and Sensory Aids Services, NY VA Medical Center, New York, New York

John Fox, CPO Supervisor of Orthotics and Prosthetics Services, Prosthetic Treatment Center, Hunter Holmes McGuire VA Medical Center, Richmond, Virginia

Allison Hickman, DO Polytrauma and Amputee Fellow, Department of Physical Medicine and Rehabilitation, Hunter Holmes McGuire VA Medical Center, Richmond, Virginia

Terry L. Kalter, MS, CP, BOCO, LPO Chief, Prosthetic Clinical Services VISN 3, Department of Veteran's Affairs, NY Harbor Healthcare Systems, New York, New York

Shane McNamee, MD Chief, Department of Physical Medicine and Rehabilitation, Hunter Holmes McGuire VA Medical Center, U.S. Department of Veterans Affairs; Assistant Professor, Department of Physical Medicine and Rehabilitation, Virginia Commonwealth University, Richmond, Virginia

Douglas Murphy, MD Associate Professor, Department of Physical Medicine and Rehabilitation, Virginia Commonwealth University; Staff Physician, Department of Physical Medicine and Rehabilitation, Hunter Holmes McGuire VA Medical Center, Richmond, Virginia

Leif Nelson, PT, DPT, ATP, CSCS Clinical Coordinator, Prosthetics and Sensory Aids Service, VA NY/NJ Healthcare System; Associate Professor, Doctor of Physical Therapy Program, Touro College, School of Health Sciences, New York, New York

Shaun O'Brien, CPO Chief of Prosthetic and Sensory Aids, Richard L. Roudebush VA Medical Center, Member of American College of Healthcare Executives, ACHE, Indianapolis, Indiana

Mary Elizabeth C. Ryan, MSPT Clinical Specialist, Physical Therapist, Department of Physical Medicine and Rehabilitation, Kessler Institute for Rehabilitation, Saddle Brook, New Jersey

Christie J. Wamsley, PT, CDE Physical Therapist, Department of Physical Medicine and Rehabilitation, Hunter Holmes McGuire VA Medical Center, Richmond, Virginia

Joseph Webster, MD Associate Professor, Department of Physical Medicine and Rehabilitation, Virginia Commonwealth University; Staff Physician, Department of Physical Medicine and Rehabilitation, Hunter Holmes McGuire VA Medical Center, Richmond, Virginia

Patty Young, MSPT, CP Amputee Rehab Coordinator, Department of Physical Medicine and Rehabilitation, Hunter Holmes McGuire VA Medical Center, Richmond, Virginia

Preface

Entering into the world of prosthetics and amputee care can appear daunting and confusing, and finding appropriate reference materials to relieve such confusion can often be difficult. *Fundamentals of Amputation Care and Prosthetics* was conceived and created to facilitate the transition to a feeling of competence for the resident physician, therapist or practitioner who has little to no background in this area. The book is designed to be carried easily within the lab coat for quick reference on issues or questions that may arise. More seasoned practitioners may also find this manual useful to refresh when providing services to amputees in the clinic or therapy setting.

Over the past decades the field of prosthetics and amputee care has made enormous gains as advances in technology have been exploited to provide prosthetic components with ever greater functionality and safety. Although concise, the book addresses the entire spectrum of relevant prosthetic parts and amputee care from quadrilateral sockets to microprocessor knees and ankle/foot complexes.

In addition to helping the practitioner prescribe the most appropriate prostheses, the book helps to troubleshoot prosthetic problems, gait issues, and medical problems. These are often tricky and subtle areas of knowledge, and our goal was to make this knowledge available in an accessible and understandable way.

The authors have been selected for their expertise and experience in this field, bringing years of practice and study to inform their chapters and offer state-of-the-art guidance. Most, if not all, have spent years teaching and thus have that added advantage as well.

All of the authors wish the readers a profitable and richly rewarding experience in using this book as they interact and work with amputees to help enrich the lives of these individuals.

Acknowledgments

The authors would like to thank Aimee St. Clair and Wayne Biggs, CPO for help with the preparation of this book. They also acknowledge Linda Droste, RN, MSN, COCN, CWCN, CCN, wound care nurse McGuire VA Medical Center, Richmond, Virginia, for assistance.

1

History of Amputation: From the Past to the Present

Shane McNamee

Reaching far back into history, mankind has attempted to compensate for the loss of limbs, through the application of prosthetic technology. While much of the history of amputee care is written into the history of war and its subsequent violence, the general population has struggled equally over time with the loss of function due to amputations from occupational injury, the damaging effects of chronic disease, and congenital limb anomalies. Great innovations have been seen throughout history with the surgical approach to non-viable limbs as well as the attempts to restore function through the application of prosthetic technology.

The history of innovation is one primarily of a response to the loss of limbs in warfare by governments struggling to successfully integrate amputees back into society. Concerted, sustained efforts have been funded by the people of the United States, Britain, Germany, Italy, Scotland, and Russia to improve the quality of the prosthetics, preparation of residual limbs, and vocationally prepare individuals for life with prosthesis. While some work has been done in the Orient throughout history, primarily in Japan, its impact upon Western Medicine has been minimal.

PRE-MODERN HISTORY

Skeletons with amputated limbs have been discovered stretching as far back as the Neolithic period. These have been discovered along with crude, stone surgical equipment. The first recorded application of a prosthetic limb was around 7000 B.C. This was recorded in the legendary Sanskrit text Rig Veda between 3,500 and 1,800 B.C. According to the text, Queen Vishpla lost a leg in battle and was fitted with an iron prosthetic limb, which allowed her to return to battle. The Greek treatise "On Joints" written around 500 B.C. describes the first known surgical approach to non-viable limbs. Its author, thought to be Hippocrates or Herodotus, prescribes amputation for gangrene below the "boundaries of blackening," once it is "fairly dead and lost its sensibility." The oldest known artificial limb in existence was unearthed in Capri, Italy in 1858. This below-the-knee wooden and copper leg was thought to date back to 300 B.C. It was unfortunately destroyed in the bombing of London during World War II.

The historical record of amputation surgery indicates that the first important threshold was crossed around the time of the birth of Christ. Surgeons, as evidenced by Celsus texts, advocated the amputation to be through healthy tissue above the gangrenous site accompanied by the ligation of vessels: ". . . between the sound and the diseased part, the flesh is to be cut through with a scalpel down to the bone, but this must not be done actually over a joint, and it is better that some of the sound part should be cut away than that any of the diseased part be left behind. When the bone is reached, the sound flesh is drawn back from the bone and undercut from around it, so that in that part also some bone is bared; bone is then to be cut through with a small saw as near as possible to the sound flesh which still adheres to it, next the face of the bone, which the saw has roughened, is smoothed down, and the skin drawn over it; this must be sufficiently loosened in an operation of this sort to cover the bone all over as completely as possible. The part where the skin has not been brought over is to be covered with lint; and over that a sponge soaked in vinegar is to be bandaged on." Heliodorus and Archigenes recommend utilizing amputation solely as a last resort and as an option for ulcers, tumors, injuries, and other deformities, around 100 A.D. Interestingly they also began to employ circumferential compression to control for blood loss. Throughout the Dark Ages, little innovation in surgical management has been noted.

The advent of gunpowder during the 14th century altered both the history of warfare and the types of military wounds. It led to a proliferation in the overall number of amputations as well as complexity in caring for the non-viable limb. A French army surgeon, Amboise Pare, reintroduced the technique of ligation, as opposed to cautery, which was advocated by Hippocrates. In the 17th and 18th centuries, advances were made with the introduction of effective tourniquets (Morel's and Petit's tourniquets) that allowed control of hemorrhage. The Parisian Petit, and later, Hey of London adapted the surgical incision from the traditional single circumferential limb incisions to more complex staged incisions of skin, muscle, fascia, and bone.

Medieval knights used artificial hands for functional means as well as for masking potential weaknesses from their opponents. The Parisian Pare designed an artificial hand "le petit Lorrain" in 1550 that had some functional components through spring loaded fingers as well as an above-the-knee-prosthesis.

The Napoleonic wars in the late 18th century brought forth plentiful opportunities for perfecting the surgical technique. Both the French surgeon Larrey and the British surgeon Guthrie challenged the long held practice of waiting the prescribed three weeks prior to amputation. They both advocated rapid amputation, which proved to lower mortality, wound infection, and issues with hemostasis. Around this time, there was a fastidious approach to the site of amputation, for the preservation of the residual limb to allow for a prosthetic interface.

STEPPING INTO MODERNITY

In the mid-18th century, two key surgical advances occurred that ushered in the modern, scientific age, for the care of those with limb loss. Ether, introduced in 1846 as an anesthetic, was a blessing obviously to the patient as well as to the surgeon. This innovation led to a less hurried approach in the surgical procedure and to more opportunities to concentrate upon, for the preparation of the limb as for an eventual prosthetic interface. This combined with the advent of antisepsis theory and practice by Lister in the late 19th century brought about the modern age of surgical amputation management. This age has been marked not only by the utilization of amputation as a lifesaving surgery, but also by a carefully executed approach, mindful of the importance of the residual limb in restoring function with eventual prosthetic fitting.

Unfortunately, the implementation of these surgical advances was sporadic throughout the American Civil War. It is estimated that 75%

of all surgeries performed in the combat theater were amputations and that more than 21,000 Union soldiers survived this procedure. Many authors documented the volume and barbarism of the field based life-saving procedures, none quite as descriptive and influential as Walt Whitman, though. Whitman, a famous author of this time, searched 40 surgical hospitals in the Washington area for his brother George. While the brothers were reunited, George suffered only a superficial facial wound. Walt was deeply moved by the horrors and human devastation he witnessed. He wrote in his notebook: "I notice a heap of amputated feet, legs, arms, hands and … human fragments, cut, bloody black and blue, swelled and sickening." Whitman volunteered as a nurse at the Armory Square Hospital in Washington D.C. Due to both his direct efforts and documentation, for the public, of the human devastation in the war, Dr. D. Willard Bliss, a prominent surgeon, claimed that "No one person who assisted in the hospitals accomplished so much good to the soldier and for the Government as Mr. Whitman."

While rudimentary prostheses were available prior to the American Civil War (1861–1865), only a small percentage of the population had access to them. The large influx of amputees and Federal (Union) and State (Confederate) funding brought about a nascent prosthetic industry in the United States. Several notable prosthetic innovations can be traced back to this time. James Edward Hanger, a Confederate lower extremity amputee, developed the "American Leg" by adding rubber bumpers to the ankle and foot. This leg made Hanger a wealthy man and it was the direct ancestor of the solid-ankle, cushioned (SACH) foot still employed today. Similar to the rapid surgical advance noted above in the 19th century, the rate of innovation of prosthetics markedly increased. This was due in part to the deployment of more careful surgical approaches as described above as well to the large number of amputees from the American Civil War. In the early 19th century, prosthetists were beginning to design upper extremity limbs in an attempt to incorporate functional joints. This includes a limb designed in 1818 by Peter Baliff, a German dentist, which is the first known limb to utilize trunk and shoulder girdle muscles for distal joint control.

THE MODERN AGE

The rapid rise of the use and the impact of the explosive ordinance in 20th century warfare markedly changed the types of injury sustained. In World War II, it was estimated that 18,000 Americans suffered an amputation from combat wounds. In 1945, the Surgeon General of the U.S. Army, Norman T. Kirk, appealed to the National Academy of Sciences (NAS) for guidance on the care of those with amputations. A conference amongst leading medical professionals and scientists was held to ascertain the state of the science. While concerted efforts had been made worldwide in the reintegration of amputees into society, the committee noted that little scientific research and development had been done in the field for amputation and prosthetic care. As a result of this effort, the NAS formed the Office of Scientific Research and Development which later changed into the Committee on Artificial Limbs (CAL), in the United States. These programs were dedicated to laying the foundation of scientific trial and advancement, which still carries on. Initially, these entities worked primarily through close linkages with medical universities and industrial laboratories. In 1947, the CAL was disbanded when the Veterans Administration was formed, and the latter took on the primary task of prosthetic innovation with the initial testing laboratory in New York City.

Philanthropy and response of the U.S. medical community led to a shift in the care of those with injuries previously considered devastating. The nascent field of care for those with amputations and prosthetics had direct ties to the advent of the field of Physical Medicine and Rehabilitation (PM&R). Dr. Howard Rusk was intimately involved in setting up programs for the combat wounded Air Force personnel at the rehabilitation center in Pawling, New York. The concept of supporting those with amputations as a whole person rather than caring for a medical condition deeply influenced the field of medicine on the whole. This program and subsequent iterations focused on the state-of-the-art technology along with "rebuilding" service members in both vocational and vocational pursuits. The success in returning to healthy lives and to full duty became the core tenets of the rapidly expanding field of PM&R.

The Korean conflict saw a steady improvement in both surgical and rehabilitation care from the foundations established during World War II. This conflict was marked by rapid troop mobilization, high casualty rates due to explosive devices, and eventually two long years of trench warfare. Advances in rapid evacuation of the injured by helicopter and implementation of aggressive vascular surgery produced a stunningly low 9% amputation rate for extremity injuries. In total, 1,120 soldiers lost limbs to traumatic amputations with a further 1,477 soldiers requiring secondary amputation surgery for mangled limbs.

The Vietnam conflict was a markedly different type of conflict, and the majority of extremity injuries were caused by small arms fire, antipersonnel mines, and booby traps such as punji sticks. This type of warfare led to an increase of 300% in lower extremity wounds from World War II and 70% from the Korean conflict. In total, 5,200 soldiers lost limbs in the Vietnam conflict. The care programs established through the Walter Reed Hospital and the Veterans Administration continued to support the care of the whole person. The shift towards the focus on residual ability rather than disability prioritized successful community re-entry. The advent of disability sports programs was seen across the nation at this time. Programs such as the adaptive skiing program at the Fitzsimons General Hospital helped amputees re-envision life after injury. These programs have direct historical links to the current adaptive sports programs for those with disability.

MODERN PROSTHETIC TECHNOLOGY

Technological explosion has accompanied the remarkable advances in the philosophical care of those with amputations. Rudimentary suspension systems have given way to innovative suction based, individually constructed socket systems. These systems allow for decreased pain, preservation of limb integrity, and functionality. Computer technology has been applied to the fitting of socket systems as well as to the successful replacement of missing joints. Computer assisted knees have now become common technology, which allows for better control, improved energy expenditure, and return to activities prohibited by mechanical technology. The quest for a functional limb has transformed to the quest for fully functioning bionic limbs.

2

Physical Exam

Shane McNamee

Like other medical conditions, an amputee's medical record should be a complete and detailed historical document. The foundation of the record is a systematic and detailed physical examination and the relevant historical elements of each particular case. The clinicians involved must approach each visit systematically with two goals in mind: (a) caring for any acute medical issues and (b) effective preparation of the limb for the utilization of a prosthetic to improve function. While a careful approach to the acute medical status is of great importance, it is the clinician's ability to prepare the limb over time that separates the experts. Only the successful management of this dynamic relationship will allow the patient to reach the highest level of function.

The goal of this chapter is to provide a systematic and comprehensive approach to meeting the goals stated above. The medical assessments above pertain to the relatively distinct phases of care that include the point prior to the amputation, the acute phase of recovery after surgery, and the period of chronic, lifelong care. Additionally, while not expressly addressed in this chapter, the clinician needs to be vigilant in the care of the contralateral limb in dysvascular patients due to the alarming rate of subsequent amputation in that limb. Patient and family education plays an important role in the preservation of the contralateral limb.

PHYSICAL EXAM

Obtaining a Useful Medical History

Past Medical History

A thorough medical history should be taken to identify medical issues that may negatively impact clinical recovery or the return of function. The underlying causes of the amputation should be clearly documented. Clinical history of pre-existing pain disorders, cardiopulmonary disease, vasculopathies, severe neurologic injury (for example, traumatic brain injury and spinal cord injury), infectious issues, and previous limb amputation should be identified due to the impact upon recovery. The clinician should address comorbidities and risk factors for amputation when possible.

Functional History

The functional history should focus upon basic functional mobility, ability to do one's activities of daily living (ADL), as well as upon the patient's environment with a particular focus on physical barriers. The examiner should gain an understanding of the patient's home environment as well as vocational and recreation environments.

Transfers. Transfers should be assessed at every visit and should approximate the patient's particular environmental issues. Therapeutic interventions are particularly effective for ameliorating these basic mobility and safety issues. The following transfers, if applicable, should be documented in the record utilizing the accepted seven-point functional independent measure (FIM):

- Bed to chair
- Seated to standing
- Chair to car
- Chair to toilet

Balance. Balance is often impaired due to the amputation as well as pre-existing alterations in the sensory system caused by peripheral nervous system diseases.

- Sitting
- Standing
- Reaching
- Moving

Mobility. The examiner should identify and assess the individual's primary method of mobility. This assists in gaining an understanding of potential barriers in function and necessary durable medical equipment that may be beneficial.

ADLs. The clinician should have an understanding of the patient's independence in basic ADL along with more complex instrumental activities.

Vascular Exam

Because vasculopathies cause or contribute to so many amputations and also create further tissue ischemia and amputation later on, a thorough vascular exam on the residual limb and intact limbs is an absolute necessity on each and every visit.

- Pulses—The presence and quality of the most distal pulses should be documented on each visit.
- Color—Cyanotic limbs may represent continued tissue ischemia due to poor arterial flow. Globally erythematous residual limbs may indicate an issue with venous drainage, that is, deep vein thrombosis (DVT), or may be a sign of infection.
- Temperature—As indicated by the color, cold limbs may indicate poor arterial supply, while warm limbs may have underlying issues with venous drainage or infection.

Skin

Acute Phase of Recovery

Providing the proper environment for the healing of wounds is necessary for optimizing outcomes. During this healing phase, the surgical site is vulnerable to infection, maceration of surrounding tissues, and dehiscence. In the post-surgical phase, the wound should be monitored daily, and the following should be documented:

- Wound approximation—The skin must be approximated for proper healing. Edema, poor surgical techniques, and tension can cause the wound edges to pull away.
- Peri-wound erythema—While some degree of erythema is expected after surgery, it can also be a sign of infection. As a rule, the erythema associated with the surgical trauma should not increase in size after 72 hours. If the erythema continues to increase in coverage, the clinician must look for other signs and symptoms of infection.

- Quality and quantity of drainage—Serosanguinous drainage is expected during the healing phase and should gradually decrease over time. Alterations in the quality of the drainage should be noted with care, with regard to pustulent or rapidly increasing bloody drainage.
- Moistness of the environment—An environment that is too wet will expose the residual limb to possible infection as well as maceration of the surrounding tissues. When the wound is too dry, the healing process is markedly restricted. Achieving the proper balance requires knowledge of wound care products and careful monitoring of the patient's individual needs.

Chronic Monitoring

During each visit, the skin at the site of the amputation should be closely examined for evidence of breakdown over bony prominences, late infection, and dehiscence of the wound. Descriptions of the following should be documented in the record:

- Surgical scar—Late dehiscence of the scar is not uncommon, and it should be monitored over time to ensure integrity. Scars that are uncommonly hard, large, or fixed to the underlying tissue may present problems with the use of a prosthesis and should be documented.
- Skin grafts—The location, healing, and the quality of tissue on skin grafts should be assessed on each visit. This includes assessing the graft site as well as the donor site.
- Moistness of the environment—Numerous types of suspension devices can lead to a very moist environment. This moisture along with the impact of loading/unloading of the prosthesis can cause significant shearing of the skin and breakdown.
- Sensation—Serial assessments should be commented on as absent, diminished, hyperesthetic, or normal.

Residual-Limb Length

The residual limb is made up of two components: bony structures and some amount of soft tissue. While the bone length should not change over time, there can be significant alterations in the amount of soft tissue. For estimating the length of the bone, the examiner should choose and use the same reference points over time. Typically. these are bony prominences in the area including the medial tibia plateau, greater trochanter of femur or humerus, and the medial epicondyle of the elbow. Increases in apparent bony length may indicate the development of heterotopic ossification.

Residual-Limb Shape

The shape of the residual limb is typically determined by the surgical technique and has great impact upon the prosthetic interface. Description of shapes include cylindrical, conical, and bulbous. Abnormalities such as "dog ears" at the surgical wound margins and adductor rolls should be documented and monitored.

Range of Motion

Joint motion can be significantly affected after amputation due to poor positioning, guarding of a painful limb, and immobility. While modern prosthetic devices can compensate for some loss in range, the maintenance of functional range in major joints is an absolute necessity for maximizing patient outcomes. On each visit, a goniometric measurement should be documented on the joints proximal to the amputation.

Neurologic Exam

- Peripheral exam—the neurologic exam should primarily focus on the integrity of the peripheral sensory system. Regardless of the cause of the amputation, the alterations in sensation in the residual limb and the site of amputation are quite common. This includes alterations in both the quality and type of sensations. In cases of vasculopathy, the contralateral limb should also be closely monitored for alterations in sensory function that leave the limb vulnerable to wounds.
- Cognitive exam—Cognitive abilities have a direct correlation to the rehabilitation and self-care of individuals, and their ability to adjust and learn new techniques. Basic bedside assessments covering the level of arousal and orientation should be documented on each visit. More comprehensive assessments with screening tools such as the Mini-Mental Status Exam and the Montreal Cognitive Assessment should be employed when potential cognitive issues are identified.

Strength

Strength should be tested over all major joints in the limbs and scored on the accepted five-point scale. Particular focus should be placed upon the joints along the kinetic chain proximal to the amputation. When a lower extremity amputation has been completed, careful testing of the hip joint must be completed, and this testing should include strength in all four planes of action (flexion, extension, abduction, and adduction) to determine eventual stability. The strength and coordination of the trunk are very important ultimately to the success in prosthetic utilization. Rapid assessment and quantification of trunk strength can be challenging, and the evaluation is most appropriately assessed during functional activities such as transfers.

CONCLUSION

The medical record should provide an accurate historical account of the patient's course of recovery after an amputation. Medical and functional recovery after amputation is by nature a dynamic process; therefore the trends in improvement, such as in function or physical findings, provide the foundation for the care of patients throughout the continuum, thereby maximizing outcomes. The clinician should approach the care of those with amputations in a stepwise manner.

APPENDIX—GUIDE FOR BEDSIDE EXAMINATION

1) Name
2) Patient Identifier
3) Date of Visit
4) Age
5) Psychosocial
    a. Living environment: ___ Alone ___ With caregivers ___ Facility
    b. Occupation
    c. Recreational activities
6) Surgical History
    a. Date(s) of amputation
    b. Reason for amputation
    c. Number of revisions and reason
7) Medical History
    a. Comorbidities: ___ Diabetes mellitus (controlled vs uncontrolled) ___ Vasculopathy ___ Residual limb infection ___ ___ Cognitive decline ___ Polytrauma
    b. Current medications
8) Patient's Prosthetic Goals
9) Functional Assessment
    a. Mobility
        i. Type of assistive device
        ii. Ambulation: ___ Non ambulatory ___ Unrestricted community ___ Household ___ Therapeutic oversight only
    b. Transfers (mark independent or physical assistance required)
        i. Bed to chair
        ii. Chair to toilet
        iii. Chair to car
        iv. Chair to stand
    c. Activities of daily living:
    d. Cognition
        i. Level of alertness: ___ Normal ___ Impaired
        ii. Orientation: ___ Person ___ Place ___ Time ___ Situation
10) Residual Limb Assessment
    a. Length (identify point of measurement origination)
    b. Shape: ___ Conical ___ Cylindrical ___ Bulbous
    c. Circumference measurements

d. Surgical Scar
    i. Intact: Y/N
    ii. Adherent to underlying tissue: Y/N
    iii. Presence of "dog ears": Y/N
    iv. Drainage: Y/N
        1. If yes describe:
e. Skin
    i. ___ Moist/macerated ___ Dry ___ Warm ___ Cool
    ii. Erythema: ___ Global ___ Focal ___ Location
    iii. Other:
f. Sensory exam: ___ Normal ___ Decreased ___ Hyperesthetic
g. Pain: describe locations and type (Musculoskeletal vs Neuropathic)
h. Joint assessment
    i. Hip
        1. Flexion: ___ ROM ___ Strength
        2. Extension: ___ ROM ___ Strength
        3. Abduction: ___ ROM ___ Strength
        4. Adduction: ___ ROM ___ Strength
    ii. Knee
        1. Flexion: ___ ROM ___ Strength
        2. Extension: ___ ROM ___ Strength
    iii. Elbow
        1. Flexion: ___ ROM ___ Strength
        2. Extension: ___ ROM ___ Strength
    iv. Shoulder
        1. Flexion: ___ ROM ___ Strength
        2. Extension: ___ ROM ___ Strength
        3. Abduction: ___ ROM ___ Strength
        4. Adduction: ___ ROM ___ Strength
        5. ___ Internal ROM
        6. ___ External ROM

3

Levels of Amputation

Douglas Murphy

METATARSAL RAY RESECTION [1–3]

1. Part removed: Metatarsal bone(s) and toe(s).
2. Indications: Congenital anomaly, chronic severe infection of a metatarsal, and gangrene such as that occurring from frostbite, subaponeurotic abscess and neoplasms.
3. Adverse consequences: The amputation leaves a narrow foot. If the first or second rays are removed then pushoff can be diminished. Fourth and fifth ray resections are better tolerated.

TRANSMETATARSAL AMPUTATION [3–6]

Amputation is carried out through the metatarsals, just proximal to the metatarsal heads [6].

1. Favorable aspects: As with other partial foot amputations, this level provides an end-bearing limb. Walking involves less work. Functional results may be better than with higher levels. It potentially provides lower morbidity and mortality when compared with results for transtibial (TT) amputations.
2. Aspects weighing against this level: The possibility of reamputation is potentially greater than with a higher level amputation chosen for the same situation.

LISFRANC AMPUTATION [1–3]

1. Level of amputation: Tarsometatarsal junction.
2. Bones removed: All phalanges and metatarsals.
3. Bones retained: Cuneiforms, cuboid, navicular, talus, and calcaneus.
4. Factors weighing against this level: The pull from the ankle plantarflexors is unopposed, and consequently, this can result in a fixed ankle plantarflexion contracture.

CHOPART AMPUTATION [1–3]

1. Level of amputation: Midtarsal joint.
2. Bones removed: Navicular, cuboid, cuneiforms, metatarsals, and phalanges.
3. Bones retained: Talus and calcaneus.
4. Factors weighing against this level: Equinovarus contracture due to the action of the calf muscles (gastrocnemius/soleus) and callus formation over the foot at its anterior and inferior portion.

PIROGOFF AMPUTATION [1–3]

1. Level of amputation: Between the tibia and calcaneus. Malleoli are removed.
2. Bones removed: Phalanges, metatarsals, cuneiforms, navicular, cuboid, talus, and part of the calcaneus.
3. Bones retained: Part of the calcaneus (with heel flap) and most of the tibia and fibula. The retained part of the calcaneus is fused to the tibia for end-bearing.
4. Factors in favor: A longer limb with lesser limp than the Symes amputation.
5. Factors weighing against this level: Failure of fusion of the calcaneus to the tibia can produce instability. The skin lying over the Achilles tendon insertion does not tolerate weight bearing well and a greater vulnerability to bursitis and ulcerations occurs. The short distance to the floor can make fitting of a prosthetic foot difficult.

BOYD AMPUTATION [1–3]

1. Location of amputation: Between the ankle mortis and calcaneus.
2. Bones removed: Phalanges, metatarsals, cuneiforms, navicular, and cuboid, part of the sustentaculum tali, talus, and cartilage

from the ankle mortise. The calcaneus is brought forward and fused into the ankle joint mortise.

3. Bones retained: Most of the calcaneus, and the tibia and fibula.
4. Features: Slightly longer than the Symes amputation. Can use the same prosthesis but may need a slight lift on the intact limb to equalize limb length. End-bearing on weight tolerant skin.

SYME AMPUTATION [1–4]

1. Level of amputation: Between the tibia and talus.
2. Bones removed: Talus, calcaneus, cuneiforms, cuboid, navicular, metatarsals, and phalanges. Parts of the malleoli are removed as well as a part of the tibia. The plane of these resections should be on a plane parallel to the floor.
3. Bones retained: The tibia and fibula are retained except for small sections of the malleoli and a small section of the distal tibia, as mentioned above.
4. Features: The heel pad and subcutaneous tissue are sutured to the distal end of the tibia for weight bearing. Weight bearing is more suitable for short distances than would be the case in a partial foot amputation, for example. Prosthetic fabrication can be challenging due to the low build height for the prosthetic foot

TRANSTIBIAL OR BELOW-KNEE AMPUTATION [2–4]

1. Level of amputation: Generally 5 to 7 inches below the joint line through the tibia and fibula.
2. Bones removed: Distal tibia and fibula and those of the foot and ankle.
3. Bones retained: Proximal tibia and fibula except for very short residual limbs when the fibula may be excised.
4. Features: Generally the fibula is sectioned 1 cm (3/8 inch) proximal to the distal tibia. The tibia is beveled in the anterior one-third.
5. Myodesis: Holes are drilled through the tibia about 1 cm proximal to the distal end. The posterior and anterior flaps are sutured to the marrow cavity.
6. Myoplasty: The flexor and extensor muscles are sutured together and to the tibial periosteum to allow the muscles to contract against resistance, and preserve blood and lymphatic return, and muscle bulk and action.

7. Ertl procedure: Periosteal flaps from the tibia and fibula are sutured together to form a bridge across the distal tibia and fibula. This bridge helps provide a pressure tolerant weight bearing surface and prevents rotation of the fibula.

Knee Disarticulation [3–5]

1. Indications: This level is chosen when there is insufficient skin coverage for a below-knee amputation (BKA) or when there is less than 4 cm or 1.5 inches of viable tibia remaining.
2. Level of amputation: This is through the knee joint.
3. Characteristics of the procedure: The patellar tendon is detached at the tibial tubercle and the cruciate ligaments are detached near the tibia. The patella is retained. The cartilage is not removed from the patella or femoral condyles. Generally, bone is not cut unless the lateral portions of the femoral condyles are shaved.
4. Factors in favor: Leaving the bone intact reduces the chances of osteomyelitis. The long femur provides a long lever arm for ambulation. Muscles that are divided in above-knee amputation (AKA) remain intact along with their attachments. Postsurgical healing is often faster and fitting of a prosthesis can occur earlier. The limb shrinks less. This level is helpful for children because the femoral epiphysis remains intact, and thus relatively normal growth of the femur can occur.
5. Factors weighing against this level: Prosthetic fitting can be difficult. Due to the increased length of the residual limb the prosthetic knee may protrude past the intact knee during sitting. Cosmetic issues can override functional advantages.

TRANSFEMORAL AMPUTATION OR ABOVE-KNEE AMPUTATION [3–5]

1. Information: Transfemoral amputation (TFA) comprises nearly 85% of all amputations. Generally, the higher the level of limb loss, the less the chance of success in rehabilitation. At least 90% of patients with BKA amputations will successfully use a prosthesis. In contrast, there is only a 25% success rate of prosthesis usage in the TFA patient.
2. Indication: This level is chosen when a BKA has a low probability of healing successfully.
3. Favorable aspects: This level has a faster rate of healing. The residual limb presents a soft tissue shell in all directions. The

time to fitting and rehabilitation often is shorter than a BKA due to generally faster healing times.

4. Factors weighing against this level: The mortality rate is greater with this procedure. There is less success with prosthetic ambulation at this level than with lower levels. The residual limb is not end-bearing. For children, the growth of the limb is impaired, and thus the limb length in adulthood may be very short. Also, with growth, the bone may push through the soft tissue.

Hip Disarticulation [3–5]

Definition and Background

Hip disarticulation involves the removal of the lower extremity from the hip joint and includes the entire femur and structures distally. A modified version consists of retaining a small portion of the proximal femur. This was a technique used to treat distal femoral osteosarcomas. Other than tumors, causative factors include trauma and severe infections. Examples of the latter are the "flesh-eating bacteria." Vascular disease and diabetic complications can result in this level of amputation as well. The procedure bears a high mortality rate and is infrequently performed. The rehabilitation challenges for this level are substantial. This level causes increased problems compared to other levels with balance in sitting, standing, walking, and with self-image.

Hemipelvectomy [3–5]

1. Indications: This procedure is often performed for malignancies of the upper thigh, hip joint, or pelvis. Further indications would include osteomyelitis of the pelvis or proximal femur.
2. Procedure: The pelvis may be separated at either the sacroiliac joint or just laterally through the ala of the ilium. The pubic bone can be sectioned 1 cm lateral to the symphysis to provide greater support to nearby organs, in part through the rectus abdominis.

Hemicorporectomy [3–5]

1. Indications: This procedure can be performed for extensive bladder cancer, rectal malignancies that involve the entire pelvis, and intractable decubiti.
2. Level of amputation: The level of transection is between the L4 and L5 vertebrae.

UPPER EXTREMITY AMPUTATIONS [3–5]

Partial Hand

Fingertip injuries have been divided into several zones to facilitate the choice of techniques for microsurgical procedures. Hirase [7] proposed zones DP-I, DP-IIA, DP-IIB, and DP-III, for this purpose. These zones have to do with the feasibility of arterial and nerve anastomosis.

The various levels of thumb amputation impair grip with varying levels of impairment (for example, 40% of hand function at the metacarpal phalangeal joint and 20% at the interphalangeal joint).

Transcarpal

Amputations at this level have the advantages of intact forearm pronation and supination as well as wrist flexion and extension. The tendons from forearm wrist flexors and extensors can be attached to the carpal bones. Cosmetic issues can detract from the advantages mentioned.

Disarticulation of the Wrist

Here the radius is separated from the carpal bones, and thus the amputee still retains supination and pronation, while at the same time having a long lever arm for lifting. This level presents cosmetic problems because the amputated side with the addition of the prosthesis can result in a longer length than the intact side. The amputee can then find this length discrepancy either intolerable or bothersome.

Transradial Amputation

A balance is necessary between preserving length for a strong lever arm and resecting enough length to allow room for prosthetic components. For the latter, the surgeon should bring the level at least 2 cm above the wrist. At the other extreme, too short a forearm residual limb will have difficulty supporting a myoelectric prosthesis due to the weight. Also, in the case of proximal level amputations, the biceps may have to be reinserted into the ulna. With a minimum of 4 to 5 cm of ulnar, active elbow flexion can be retained.

Elbow Disarticulation

Elbow disarticulation presents conflicts between opposing functional concerns. The length and presence of the humeral epicondyles allow a greater lever arm, and enhance suspension and rotational control. However, the extra length disallows the incorporation of a prosthetic elbow. Instead, elbows with external hinges have been specifically designed, and these present cosmetic issues for some users.

Transhumeral

The surgeon attempts to preserve as much length of the humerus as possible. However, in order to accommodate prosthetic components, the distance from the tip of the olecranon to the distal end of the resected humerus should be at least 10 cm. The biceps and triceps should be firmly attached to the bone, if the length permits. If at all possible, the insertion of the deltoid into the humerus should be kept in order for the amputee to maintain active control of the shoulder. Resection of the humerus very close to the glenohumeral joint results in a level that is functionally similar to a shoulder disarticulation. However, its advantage includes maintaining the contour of the shoulder. For transections through the humeral neck, arthrodesis should be included in order to prevent abduction contractures. Even a small degree of humeral retention permits better suspension of the prosthesis. Very short transhumeral amputations can be considered a modified shoulder disarticulation.

Shoulder Disarticulation

The deltoid is used for padding and coverage. If for some reason the deltoid cannot be used, then the anterior, posterior, or axillary skin is employed. Additionally, the acromion and coracoid process may have to be decreased. For the acromion, usually the distal third is removed.

Scapulothoracic Amputation

This level may be required in cases of malignancy, necrotizing fasciitis, or trauma. The entire arm, the scapula, and generally, most of the clavicle are removed. This level creates substantial cosmetic concerns for the individual.

REFERENCES

1. May BJ. *Amputations and Prosthetics: A Case Study Approach,* 2nd ed. F.A. Davis Company; 2002.
2. Sanders GT. *Lower Limb Amputations: A Guide to Rehabilitation*. F.A. Davis Company; 1986.

3. Smith DG, Michael JW, Bowker JH. *Atlas of Amputations and Limb Deficiencies: Surgical, Prosthetic, and Rehabilitation Principles*, 3rd ed. American Academy of Orthopedic Surgeons; 2004.
4. Lenhart MK, ed in chief, Pasquina Paul F, Cooper RA, eds. *Textbooks of Military Medicine: Care of the Combat Amputee.* Office of the Surgeon General at TMM publications; 2009, pp. 117–191.
5. Lusardi MM, Nielsen CC. *Orthotics and Prosthetics in Rehabilitation*. 2nd ed. Elsevier; 2007, pp. 563–592.
6. Brown ML, Tang W, Patel A, Baumhauer JF. Partial foot amputations in patients with diabetic foot ulcers. *Foot Ankle Int*. Sep 2012;33(9):707–716.
7. Hirase Y. Salvage of fingertip amputated at nail level: New surgical principles and treatments. *Ann Plastic Surg.* Feb 1997;38(2):151–157.

4

Pre- and Post-Operative Care: Readiness for Fitting

Christie J. Wamsley

PRE- AND POST-OPERATIVE CARE OF THE LOWER EXTREMITY AMPUTEE

The decision to amputate a limb, whether it is secondary to vascular disease, trauma, or neoplasm is forever life changing, for not only the individual, but their family as well. An attempt to salvage a limb sometimes in itself can become burdensome, requiring months or years of wheelchair bound status, continuous pain, wound vacs (vacuum-assisted closures), multiple debridements, and time consuming and costly clinical follow-up.

Patients and their families sometimes buy into having an amputation when they can no longer pursue their life's interests, whether it is working, family activities, household chores, hunting, fishing, or just out of a desire to live life without pain.

The team approach is the critical element in setting the tone for having a positive outcome and promoting the total rehabilitation process from acute care to evaluation for prosthetic fitting. Emphasis should be placed on gaining the patient and the family's confidence in regard to surgical technique, timeliness of the surgery, avoidance of revisions, and providing the opportunity for future prosthetic consideration. A positive outcome is often determined when open lines of communication are established during pre-op, post-op, and early pre-prosthetic periods. This is an opportunity when expectations are discussed, questions answered, goals discussed, and the plan of care outlined. A discussion of the expected plan of care can alleviate anxiety, enhancing compliance in the acute care environment, which is required throughout the entire rehab process. It is critical that all team members are sensitive to the patient's ability to cope with the loss of limb and their ability to start preparing for life with or without a prosthesis.

Pre-Operative Care

A pre-op evaluation is the ideal opportunity to predict mobility outcome in one year based on the knowledge of peri-operative factors. Appropriate discussions prior to amputation enhance the consent process and improve treatment planning. The informed consent process provides legalistic protection for the physician and hospital, facilitates quality patient–physician interaction, provides an opportunity for shared decision making, and outlines relative risks and expected outcomes. Considerations are mortality, functional outcome, and healing of the surgical site. The goal is to enlighten and educate the patient. It is important to convey that there is never the right level of amputation, stressing the "value of life" even if in a wheelchair.

Early involvement of a peer visitor might provide the patient insight and understanding of the healing and rehab process, provide coping strategies, and provide assurance that there is support available throughout the entire process. The Amputee Coalition of America has a database of trained, certified volunteers available to assist with this coping process. The mission of peer visitors is to reinforce that everyone's experience is unique, to provide encouragement, and to provide a supportive and understanding listener.

Supportive counseling by Psychology or Mental Health may be required to validate patients' anxieties, assist with involving their support system, and provide coping strategies through the entire process, especially in dealing with the immediate loss of limb.

Social work intervention may assist early in making the patient and their family aware of community resources/veterans' assistance programs and resources, and assistance with financial concerns, defining available home care services, and discussing disposition options, whether it is inpatient rehabilitation, skilled nursing facility, palliative/hospice care, or home.

Post-Operative Care

The major priorities of post-operative care for the amputee are straightforward. They are the promotion of wound healing, pain control for conditions such as phantom limb sensation/pain, volume control, functional mobility, continued emotional support, education, and discharge planning. This is considered the healing and protective phase. Inpatient stay ranges from 5 days to 2 weeks depending on the reason for amputation, the patient's age, comorbidities, pain management, disposition, and post-op complications.

Recognition of Post-Operative Complications

Immediately post-op, the focus is on the prevention of post-op complications. The early recognition of possible post-op complications such as deep venous thrombosis (DVT), pulmonary embolus (PE), arrhythmias, congestive heart failure (CHF), sepsis, renal failure, infection, and hematoma could not only effect overall prognosis, but rehab potential as well. Complications may occur in any amputee, though the typical dysvascular patient may present more obvious risks. The typical patient is over 60 years old, a smoker, diabetic with cardiac disease, peripheral vascular disease, chronic kidney disease, chronic obstructive pulmonary disease (COPD), a history of alcohol abuse, and post-traumatic stress disorder.

Chart Review

The chart review of the new amputee is paramount to ensure all factors are considered when initiating the rehab process. First, the weight and the recent weight trends, as well as body mass index (BMI) should be reviewed to assess the patient's overall health status prior to the amputation. Next, labs, such as PT/INR (prothrombin time/international normalized ratio), WBC (white blood cell count), HCT (hematocrit) and HgB (hemoglobin) are reviewed to ensure the patient will be appropriate for participation in exercise at that time. If the patient is diabetic, the blood glucose level as well as the Hemoglobin A-1C should be checked prior to participation in physical therapy. The patient's medication list should be assessed to give further insight into the past medical history based on pharmacologic involvement in their overall health. Vascular study results should be checked to assess the overall circulation health of the remaining limb. Finally, the assessment of use of tobacco, alcohol and substance abuse should be considered as this puts the patient at risk for poor healing. Past medical compliance is relevant and may have a direct effect on the outcome providing insight regarding risk reduction interventions.

History

In order to determine the level of care and ability to transition to home, certain social considerations must be reviewed. To start, the patient's home environment and potential barriers to mobility must be considered and an assessment of durable medical equipment (DME) should be made. The amount of caregiver and family support must also be assessed as the patient will require assistance that is consistent and reliable. Another factor, the mode of travel in the community, is important to factor into the evaluation as the patient will need to have accessibility to the community in order to perform tasks such as grocery shopping, attend doctors visits and prosthetic fabrication, if appropriate. Finally, the premorbid level of mobility should be a consideration in order to assist in goal setting and to ascertain the true potential for the patient to walk with or without a prosthesis.

It is important to assess the patient's cognition/mental acuity (mini-mental examination) initially, and on follow-up visits, determine their safety awareness, discuss their fears and anxieties, note their ability to follow commands, and determine their suited style of learning. A discussion of the patient's goals and the evaluation of emotional well-being should also occur.

Evaluation—ROM, Strength, and Balance

Range of motion (ROM), strength, and balance can be evaluated during functional activities at the bedside by observing activities of daily living (ADL) during co-treatment sessions with physical and occupational therapists, and nursing. Useful information can be gathered by observing a patient's bed mobility, balance during dressing activities, bladder and bowel regimen, and handling of the residual limb.

Proper positioning post-op is critical initially as pain may result in a protective flexion withdrawal pattern without the sensory feedback of weight bearing activities. Flexion contractures can prolong the time to prosthetic fit or even result in the inability to fit a patient with prosthesis.

The most frequently seen contracture for the transtibial (TT) amputee is a knee flexion contracture, which can be prevented by donning a knee immobilizer immediately post-op or intra-operatively. The immobilizer is protective and helps to prevent trauma to the distal end of the residual limb. Such trauma can cause an ecchymosis or wound dehiscence, and thus potentially could prolong a hospital stay and delay the time to prosthetic fit. Air splints, bi-valve casts, and orthoplast splints are other options. Prolonged wheelchair sitting with the knee flexed further facilitates a contracture, which might be avoided by simply placing the residual limb on a sliding board supported on an elevating leg rest. A commercial amputee prop that is level with the wheelchair cushion can position the amputated limb in an ideal manner. The mechanism is adjustable and swings away to permit a smaller wheelchair turning radius. A limitation in hamstring range in the TT amputee may result in posterior pelvic tilt and sacral sitting with increased risk of skin breakdown and mechanical low back pain with prosthetic gait.

Frequent contractures seen in the transfemoral amputee include hip flexion, external rotation, and abduction. A pillow placed laterally alongside the residual limb will facilitate neutral position. Frequent prone positioning for the TT and transfemoral amputee is encouraged early in the acute phase. The Thomas test can be used to evaluate the tightness of a hip flexion contracture for both TT and transfemoral amputees. This same position can be used for low load stretching of hip flexion contractures.

Skin

All boney prominences should be examined. If a patient has a sacral decubitus ulcer, sheer should be avoided by not raising the head of the bed over 30°. Frequent turning using positioning wedges and a specialty mattress should be used if posture cannot be altered. Wheelchair push-ups for pressure relief should be performed every hour.

Inspection of the remaining foot is paramount for the diabetic amputee, given that statistics state that there is a 50% increase in incidence of amputation of the contralateral limb within four years after the primary amputation. Vascular amputees should be provided early information regarding this grave statistic and informed that the chance of achieving a functional gait as a bilateral amputee is less of a reality considering the energy cost and prolonged time required for fitting and gait training. Wheelchair mobility may become more practical since it can be faster and more energy conserving. Neurologic testing should include the measurement of protective sensation using a 10-g Semmes–Weinstein monofilament (representing the pressure threshold to protect against ulceration), evaluation of the Achilles and patella reflexes, and vibratory, temperature, and proprioception sensation. The distal pulses in both legs should be compared through palpation. Observation might reveal a variety of structural deformities such as prominent metatarsal heads, Charcot foot deformity, bunions, corns, calluses, onychomycosis, hammertoes, dryness with maceration, limited toe and ankle range, and past amputation of toes. Ulceration along the medial and lateral aspects of the feet might be indicative of shoes that are too tight while plantar ulceration may indicate repetitive pressures over prominent metatarsal heads in an intrinsic minus foot. If there are risk factors, and if the remaining foot is dysvascular, then gait should be discouraged, with standing limited to transfers and balance activities. Preventive measures are often overlooked in the acute care setting where the patient might benefit from a referral to a pedorthist and a podiatrist. The patient should be instructed to avoid barefoot walking even in the home setting, perform daily foot inspections with an inspection mirror, and apply appropriate routine foot care for managing xerosis, calluses, and nail care. Appropriate shoe rotation should occur. The shoes at the bedside should be inspected for wear and proper fit. Impaired vision may be a barrier to early recognition of ulceration requiring referral to appropriate resources.

The residual limb incision should be evaluated for tissue integrity and signs of inflammation. Girth measurements should be tracked every 4 cm. Fitting with a prosthesis can be considered when the distal residual limb circumference is equal to or not more than a quarter inchlarger than the circumference of the proximal portion of the residual limb. Limb length should be documented with the ischial tuberosity used as a proximal landmark for the transfemoral amputation and the tibial tubercle for the TT amputee. With increased limb loss, energy expenditure increases, and velocity decreases when the amputee is fit and is walking with a prosthesis.

Transfers

The effects of prolonged bed rest may contribute to deconditioning resulting in cardiopulmonary risks with even the lowest level of activity. The practitioner should work with the patient and their family to encourage the patient to work to become independent with transfers, including bed mobility without the use of bed rails, trapeze bars or bed controls for positioning. The perceived level of exertion and dyspnea should be noted when performing bed mobility. Vitals should be monitored to avoid episodes of orthostatic hypotension or autonomic changes in the diabetic patient. Caution should be taken with the patient with elevated blood pressure at rest, lack of systolic blood pressure response with increased workload or tachycardia at rest. Finally, an active stretching and warm-up regimen should be performed prior to sitting at the edge of the bed and prior to standing.

The method of transfer (sliding board, squat pivot, or lift aide), degree of assist, and safe wheelchair preparation should be communicated to the nursing staff and family. The wheelchair should be an appropriate fit. Those patients who have bilateral lower limb amputations will require a wheelchair with an amputee axle plate to ensure their center of mass is repositioned over the center axle of the wheelchair. Anti-tippers are a solution, though they make curb negotiation and access of ramps difficult. Offset axle plates increase the work of propulsion and may have limitations in shoulder ROM, which may impose additional difficulties. Removable arm rests are a necessity for sliding board transfers and allow the wheelchair to move closer to some objects such as tables. Progression of transfer activities should include chair to toilet, chair to tub, vehicle transfers, and floor transfers. Floor mobility, including scooting and bumping up/down stairs may become a necessity in an unramped home. Limitations in strength, ROM, and deconditioning in the elderly or medically complex amputee may present difficulties. Commercial cushions are available to protect the ischii and sacrum from trauma with floor transfers and mobility.

Accessibility of all doors in the home should be discussed and options such as widening doors, removing the door molding/frame, or the removal of doors for non-ambulatory or bilateral amputees should also be reviewed. The use of a travel chair or the removal of push rims may aid in gaining access to bathrooms or negotiating narrow hallways. Durable medical equipment needed for safe tub transfers should be prescribed and the wearing of a swim shoe should be encouraged to protect the sound foot and avoid a fall.

Single limb balance using an assistive device is introduced to allow the amputee to learn how to compensate for the loss of the limb and shifting the center of mass over the sound limb. Good static and challenged standing balance will instill confidence with transfers and allow progression to a hop-to-gait as permitted for short distances in areas not accommodating a wheelchair. The ability to advance gait on the sound limb is reflective of the patient's ability to control the prosthetic limb in stance phase. Strength, balance, and proprioception are all components of this skill. Not all patients will be suitable for prosthetic fitting. Factors to consider for this decision would include pre-operative ambulatory status, ability to ambulate in the parallel bars, and response to current workloads. It requires more energy to walk with a walker without a prosthesis than with a prosthesis.

Compressive Dressings

Many options exist for post-operative dressing. The choice depends primarily on physician preference, but other considerations that can influence the decision are healing potential, patient compliance, surgical technique, and level of amputation. It is critical to manage post-op edema and protect the incision. Compression dressings can assist with pain control, desensitization, increasing circulation, and reducing phantom limb pain/sensation. Some of the choices are as follows:

1. Soft dressings such as a gauze, soft padding, and co-band or ace bandages available in varying widths (2, 4, or 6 inches) are

worn 24 hours a day and are most commonly used early on in the dysvascular amputee. Care must be taken to avoid wrapping, so that a tourniquet effect will not occur. An elastic stockinette is another substitute used over soft gauze that provides compression and holds dressings in place.

2. Rigid dressings and immediate post-operative prosthesis (IPOP) applied immediately after surgery maintain the knee in extension in the TT amputee. There is risk of increased pressure and a possible delay in the identification of wound care problems. In IPOP, padding is placed over boney prominences and other modifications to allow weight bearing with a prosthesis. These types of dressings are rarely used in the vascular patient.
   a. Shorter time periods from amputation to prosthetic fit have been documented with the use of semi-rigid and rigid dressings.
3. Removable custom rigid dressings fashioned out of plaster or polyethylene function as dressings and also provide protection to the residual limb. They can be removed for skin inspection. The ability to don/doff socks provides an introduction to initial prosthetic wearing, when sock adjustment is required for optimum fit. When as many as 15 sock ply are required to maintain contact and fit, then generally speaking, another removable dressing should be fabricated. A TT amputee is able to progress to limited distal weight bearing on a stool, 12 to 15 days after surgery or when the incision is not at risk of dehiscence. This dressing is difficult to fabricate when there is an exceptionally bulbous distal residual limb and can be uncomfortable in donning/doffing. Often a commercial shrinker is used during non-wearing times such as during sleep for comfort or they can be used in conjunction with the removable rigid dressing. There are commercial non-custom versions made of plastic, which are secured with Velcro; they fit but are not ideal.
4. Commercial shrinkers are preferred in some institutions over traditional ace wrapping. They require little skill in donning and can be pulled over the residual limb with a donning tube for those with limited hand dexterity or excessive residual limb pain, provide more consistent pressure, and are available for both TT and transfemoral amputees. They are usually initiated once the surgical incision is healed (usually 10 days or when the incision is no longer at risk). A nylon sheath can be used as an interface to avoid shear and protect the incision. The use of tubigrip has become common practice for compression as the patient will don the

tubigrip shrinker with a long first layer and then double the tubigrip at the distal-most portion of the limb to create venous return.

a. The consistent wearing of shrinkers whenever the prosthesis is not in place is often necessary for edema control during the first year after the amputation. Seasoned prosthetic wearers may still require the use of a shrinker to maintain prosthetic fit secondary to fluctuations in circumference such as in the end-stage renal disease (ESRD) patient or those with other medical conditions such as CHF. Prosthetic wearers sometimes choose to wear the liner instead of a shrinker to maintain the circumference needed for donning the prosthesis.

Skin Care, Scar Management, and Wound Care

Often sutures and staples are left in place in the dysvascular amputee up to one month post-operatively. If staples are removed, steri strips are applied and allowed to remain in place until they separate and fall off. It is important to mobilize the scar once wound healing is complete. The prime time to attempt to mobilize the incision line and prevent adhesions to the underlying tissue is when the scar is not yet mature. Pressure is applied above and below the incision line mobilizing the incision. Olive oil, cocoa butter, and vitamin E cream are some of the agents used to facilitate massage and prevent dryness. Once the prosthetic wearing is initiated, an adherence along the suture line could result in skin breakdown delaying ambulation. Sensory testing of the residual limb should be carried out as relevant in prosthetic consideration and the type of insert. Open wounds may require consultation with a wound care nurse. A vacuum assisted wound closure device may facilitate early closure and prosthetic fit.

Good nutrition is essential for all wound healing. Adequate nutrition for anabolism requires an Albumin level of at least 3.0 and a prealbumin level of 20. A multi-vitamin with minerals is suggested for wound healing. The practitioner should be aware of any wound drainage in excess as loss of fluid from the wound/incision site would put the patient at risk for dehydration.

Another approach to wound healing might be electrical stimulation, which facilitates healing by increasing capillary density, improving tissue oxygenation, and aiding granulation tissue formation and fibroblastic activity.

Bioelectrical activity is normally present in skin, but during tissue injury, the electrical field is diminished and cells have difficulty migrating for tissue repair. The synthesized electrical activity generates a signal to the cells, which is essential to the cascade reaction to achieve wound healing.

Electrical stimulation has bacteriostatic properties that help to reduce the number of bacteria by generating galvanotaxis in the wound. Conditions that might be present in the amputee population, which may be indicated for treatment with this modality are the following:

1. Recalcitrant stage II, III, and IV pressure ulcer
2. Arterial ulcer
3. Neuropathic ulcer
4. Venous stasis ulcer.

Exercise

Early mobility has been shown to improve functional outcomes, promote independence, decrease mortality rates, and reduce the length of stay for individuals with lower extremity amputation. Muscle strength is lost faster than gained with strengthening exercises.

The ability to transfer, stand, and propel a wheelchair requires baseline functional strength. Muscle strengthening should be initiated as soon as the aerobic condition provides adequate peripheral oxygenation before and during mobility by monitoring vital signs, monitoring perfusion in the lower extremities, and monitoring rate of perceived exertion/rate of perceived dyspnea (RPE/RPD).

Exercises specific to strengthening the sound limb are crucial, considering the overuse demands placed on it and the possibility of the extremity buckling during transfers and attempted ambulation resulting in a fall. Lower extremity amputees must maximize strengthening potential as they lack the ankle strategies and have impaired hip strategies secondary to the lack of somatosensory input and must depend on intact vision and lumbo-pelvic stabilization.

An initial exercise regimen may consist of simple anti-gravity exercises, isometrics, and ankle pumps progressing to resisted closed kinetic chain exercises. Wheelchair propulsion and a wheelchair aerobic regimen will allow patients a way for independently exercising and will incorporate practice in functional activities as well. The gold standard exercise for both transfemoral and TT amputees is prone lying, which promotes extension and combats hip flexion contractures acquired from prolonged wheelchair sitting. Patients should be able to advance to alternate arm/leg lifts and progress to activities on elbows. Simple towel rolls or pillows can be used for resisted hip/knee extension and abduction/adduction of the hip in supine, side lying, and prone postures.

Theraband can be a way to provide resistance supine and seated. All of these pre-prosthetic exercises can be performed in the home care setting with repetitions and sets increased according to the frequency, intensity and time (FIT) principle and patient's tolerance. The post-op exercise regimen should be tailored to the level of amputation and should consider any precautions related to the surgical procedure. The goal is to provide a basic functional exercise regimen that can be performed independently and with carry-over in the next setting allowing progression to Phase II rehab where a more vigorous and pre-prosthetic regimen can be implemented.

Core strengthening (lumbo-pelvic–hip complex) is a focal point not to be ignored. It could be initiated by having the patient contract the lower abdomen achieving neutral spine. The transversus abdominis and multifidi can be further strengthened with bridging, leg circles, hands over head, and alternate hands on knees. Neutral spine progression to seated and standing postures incorporating Kegels allows enhanced kinesthetic awareness. Adequate core strength provides a base for upper and lower extremity activities as well as prevents chronic low back pain and gait dysfunction with later prosthetic training.

At the appropriate moment, the upper body ergometer (UBE) provides good cardio-pulmonary fitness, and the results serve as a predictor of prosthetic success. The Nu-step allows exercise of the upper extremities and sound limb, allowing increased activity with a lower perceived level of exertion.

Phantom Pain, Phantom Limb Sensation, and Residual Limb Pain

Eighty five percent of amputees will experience one or all three types of pain or abnormal sensation at one time or another, with the greatest number experienced during the first year post-operatively. The cause of residual limb pain may be a neuroma, improper wrap, entrapped scar, alteration in blood flow, insufficient nutrition, or disrupted sleep pattern. Preferably, the patient's pain should be managed prior to any physical activity, wound care, or management of the residual limb, and rated by the visual analog pain scale. Every effort should be provided to minimize and control pain allowing maximal mobility and rehabilitation during this short inpatient hospital stay.

Phantom limb pain occurs within the non-existent portion of the limb and is often described as a dull ache, burning, knife-like, electrical shock, or a sensation that the limb is being ripped off. Provocation might include dressing changes, stress or other irritants, or cold.

Phantom sensation is described as if the extremity is still present and patients may describe symptoms of itching, wetness, generalized discomfort, and heaviness.

Pain assessment should begin pre-operatively with treatment through all phases of rehabilitation. Treatment may include pharmacological treatment including anticonvulsants, antidepressants, nonsteroidal anti-inflammatory drugs (NSAIDS), opioids, lidoderm patches, and topical analgesics such as capsaicin cream allowing active rehab participation. Medication should be provided prior to dressing changes and rehab sessions. It is relevant for the therapist to be aware of the side effects of medications as side effects might include orthostatic hypotension, lethargy, disinterest, and cognitive impairment.

A non-pharmacological approach might include an attempt to desensitize by tapping, stimulation with varied textured fabrics, transcutaneous electrical neuromuscular stimulation (TENS), acupuncture, and bio-feedback. Mirror box therapy is a cortical restructuring attempt recreating a body image by performing therapeutic exercise, using a mirror to view the reflection of an anatomical limb in the space occupied by the phantom limb.

Outcome Measures

There are a variety of standardized tests and measures that may be beneficial in determining the degree of social support, defining equipment needs, and predicting prosthetic fit.

The Functional Independent Measure (FIM) should be performed early in the post-op period and prior to discharge. It is not a good predictor of success with regard to prosthetic fit and does not fully capture functional changes with the progression of therapy, secondary to the ceiling effect. It is a standard outcome measure for amputees, especially for patients with additional medical complexity such as traumatic brain injury (TBI) and stroke.

The Amputee Mobility Predictor (AMP) is considered to be a valid outcome measure with and without prosthesis and can be performed in 15 minutes or less. It correlates with the 6-minute walk as a predictor of prosthetic success. It is always of value to access patients for what they can do rather than what they cannot do.

There are other suggested outcome measures more appropriate for later phases of amputee rehabilitation.

Discharge Planning and Summary

Prior to discharge, patients should be provided with written guidelines including a home exercise regimen, skin care, residual limb care, listing of community resources, and follow-up appointments with the surgeon and rehab disciplines.

Patients should be provided with the appropriate wound care supplies, topical wound care medications, nutritional information, and the needed durable medical equipment.

The length of acute care stay is dictated by multiple factors including amputation level, wound healing, complications post-op, cognition, social support, and home accessibility. Home health referral may be needed to address short-term rehab needs until the transition to outpatient rehabilitation, at which time the patient is independent with ADL and mobility. The patient usually undergoes a more dynamic pre-prosthetic/conditioning regimen preparing for prosthetic fit and training. An introduction to adaptive and recreational activities for lifelong cardio-pulmonary fitness, outpatient cardiac rehab once fit with prosthesis, driver's training with vehicle modification, vocational rehabilitation, and modification of patient's work station for reintegration into the community may be appropriate in the next phase of care.

If the transition home is inappropriate and the medical and surgical needs of the patient have not been met, an inpatient rehabilitation stay may be appropriate. There should be defined rehab goals related to function and transition home, and the patient should be able to tolerate 3 hours of rehab daily. Transfer to a skilled nursing facility (SNF) may be needed, when home health services are not sufficient for independent living, additional rehab is needed, or skilled surgical and medical needs arise.

The patient should be reminded that lifelong follow-ups may be needed for ongoing prosthetic management and care. Scheduled appointments are established for 1, 3, and 6 months, together within annual follow-up visit.

BIBLIOGRAPHY

Browken JH, Pfeifer MA. *Levine and O'Neal's The Diabetic Foot*, 7th ed. Mosby, Inc; 2008.

Luardi MM, Neilson CC. *Orthotics and Prosthetics in Rehabilitation*, 2nd ed. Saunders; 2007.

PT AMP Protocol. Washington D.C.: Walter Reed Hospital; 2009.

Standard of Care: LE Amputation. Brigham and Women's Hospital; 2001.

VA/DoD Clinical Practice Guidelines for Rehabilitation of Lower Extremity Amputation, Department of Veterans Affairs, Department of Defense; 2008. http://www.healthquality.va.gov, https://www.gmo.amedd.army.mil

5

Rehab Post Surgery

Mary Elizabeth C. Ryan and Patty Young

REHAB WITH A TEMPORARY PROSTHESIS

The excitement of learning to use a new prosthetic limb can be overwhelming. Although the new amputee may have many questions and queries, the practitioner must emphasize to the patient that the initial prosthetic training requires time, energy, and patience, and is not an easy or quick process. It is important for the practitioners working with the patient to provide the new wearer with both written instructions and demonstration to ensure that the amputee has all the necessary information when going home. The following factors should be emphasized as the focus of their rehab with their temporary prosthesis.

Skin Checks

Practitioners are encouraged to initiate training with an in-depth discussion and education session strongly emphasizing the importance of skin checks. The patient needs to be reminded that the residual limb is not accustomed to pressures of both perpendicular and vertical forces, and therefore should become very familiar with every aspect of their residuum, including the color, shape, incision line, bony prominences, and any areas of irregularities. This population of people is often affected by comorbidities and secondary impairments such as decreased sensation, visual deficits, decreased circulation, compromised skin integrity, and possible cognitive involvement contributing to the importance of close monitoring and individualized attention.

Inspection should start with the incision line. An inspection mirror is an important tool to use as well as detailed education for the family member to ensure thorough inspection of not only the residual limb but also the sound limb. The scar and the tissue surrounding the scar should be mobile to decrease frictional forces within the socket. If the scar is adhered below the surface, the patient should be instructed in scar mobilization technique in order to prevent blisters and skin breakdown. After inspecting the incision line, the skin around bony prominences, such as the distal end of the tibia or fibular head in the transtibial and the distal femur on the transfemoral should be inspected before and after removal of the prosthesis to affirm that the skin has not had changes other than a slight redness to the area after wearing the prosthesis. Finally, an inspection of the soft tissue areas of the limb (posterior tissue of the transtibial and the groin area of the transfemoral) should be performed noting any areas of redness, irritation, or blanching. The definition of undesirable redness in prosthetic wearing is any redness that lasts longer than 10 minutes or redness over bony prominences. Acceptable redness lasts less than 10 minutes and is even in color and located in areas where desirable pressure is required for residual limb control within the socket. The desirable areas of weight bearing and pressure in the transtibial socket are along the tibial crest, at the patellar tendon bar, along the fibular shaft, broadly in the area of the medial tibial flare, and along the proximal tissue. In the transfemoral socket, there is expected redness along the brim, especially on the ischial tuberosity and the anterior medial wall, and there may be redness generally along the soft tissue on the mid-to-distal residuum. Again, it is important to notice areas of redness lasting longer than 10 minutes, and areas with noted skin tearing or ulceration should be communicated to the physical therapist and the prosthetist immediately.

Skin checks are imperative to prevent skin breakdown while integrating increased weight bearing through the socket. While acclimating to the shape of the socket and pressures on the limb, skin checks are performed frequently during the initial training and should happen throughout the day. These skin checks may influence the wearing schedule and the number of sock ply the patient wears in order to optimize the fit of the socket. A common pattern for wearing time in order to best acclimate the residuum to the pressures of the socket is to start with a minimum time of 15 minutes with the prosthesis on, followed by 30 minutes out of the socket; for example, 15 minutes on, 30 minutes off, 15 minutes on, 30 minutes off, etc. The emphasis should be on skin checks when the prosthesis is removed. The progression in wearing time should be increased by 15 minutes each time the socket is donned every other day, thus increasing the "on time" and later decreasing the "off time." The practitioner should work closely with the amputee in determining an appropriate wearing schedule as other factors may affect prosthetic use such as residual limb shape and predisposition to skin breakdown. This will take time to build up a tolerance to wearing the prosthesis and should be followed strictly by the patient to ensure that the time is spent adjusting to the socket.

Sock Ply Management

Sock ply management tends to be the most challenging aspect of the learning process in initial prosthetic training but is most imperative for prevention of skin breakdown and to ensure good suspension. It seems the hardest part of learning about sock ply management is the lack of comparable experience in one's life prior to the amputation, so learning and truly understanding when to add a sock ply and when to remove a sock ply is a foreign concept. To explain to a new wearer the socket should feel as snug each time it is donned as it is the *very first time* the leg is worn is a very difficult concept for these individuals to internalize since oftentimes sensation is compromised due to secondary complications. Sock ply should be added and removed one ply at a time, not one sock at a time, and this should be reinforced over and over again. It seems, with confidence, a new wearer will add socks without taking into account the ply each sock provides to the fit and comfort of the prosthesis.

It is at this time, the initial stage of prosthetic wearing education, time that the therapist and the prosthetist should discuss the reasons for volume fluctuation in the residuum. Volume fluctuation tends to be a difficult concept to grasp for new amputees. The fluctuation is constant and the fit of the socket is forever changing from the moment of initial donning throughout the amputee's lifetime. Factors affecting volume in the residual limb include muscle atrophy or hypertrophy, weight loss/gain, medical side effects from dialysis such as fluid retention and the amount of time the amputee spends in a weight bearing position. Weight shifting during standing and walking creates a pumping mechanism causing changes in volume in the residual limb.

Since compromised sensation is so common to the general population of prosthetic wearers, the provider can provide guidance by emphasizing a few general nuances with donning that may provide the wearer with clues as to the need for more or less sock ply. The ease with which the prosthesis is donned is the first indication of the need for adjusting the sock ply; if the individual is able to slide the limb in without any resistance, this may indicate a need for adding a sock ply but if the limb is unable to fit completely into the socket, then sock plies may need to be removed one ply at a time until the donning process is easier. Another hint to cue a wearer as to the proper position of the residuum within the socket is through the alignment of specific bony landmarks with areas on the socket; such as the patellar tendon bar of the socket coordinating with the area of the wearer's patellar tendon or the fibular head corresponding with the fibular head relief. Finally, with a pin suspension, the number of "clicks" heard when sliding into the lock mechanism in the donning process can give a new wearer a sense of where the residuum is falling within the socket; for example, if at the initial delivery of the prosthesis the new wearer hears only 4 clicks and the fit is ideal, but at a later time, the wearer hears 12 clicks, this may indicate the need for one or more sock plies.

The general rule in sock ply management is to know that one ply is 2 mm of thickness and refers to one strand of thread. Each ply added will change the way the socket fits but it should be noted that the change in fit will be universal and not point specific; in other words, if you have areas that tend to be bony prominences such as the fibular head, adding a three-ply sock adds an extra 6 mm and will apply undo pressure possibly causing pain. An alternative to traditional, full-length prosthetic socks are half socks and compensator socks. The benefit to using a half sock is the length of the sock will address only what is at the distal end of the limb and not add bulk to the bony anatomy at the proximal areas such as the patella, tibial plateau or the ischium in the transfemoral socket. A compensator sock is used to provide a tapered fit so there is thickness at the distal end while maintaining coverage of the bony anatomy proximally.

Specific areas of redness can be indicative of either too many socks or too few socks although these examples can also pertain to alignment issues. For example, if a person is exhibiting redness on the inferior limb and the distal most point of the tibia, the assumption is that the individual is falling too far into the socket and "bottoming out," thereby requiring more sock ply to lift the residuum off the bottom of the socket. Another example is when a residuum has redness along bony prominences that were not red before. If these red marks are consistent along all bony prominences and are below the bony prominences, this implies that the residuum is not sitting into the socket as it should be and the wearer has too much sock ply on. Conversely, if the red marks are over the bony prominences, the wearer may be too far in the socket and this indicates pistoning up and down of the residuum within the socket.

Donning/Doffing

Donning the prosthesis should be done in a methodical way each time the limb is worn. The therapist should take the time to ensure that the education of the patient and their family members is thorough and succinct so as to minimize confusion. Written instructions as well as illustrations may be helpful, but emphasis should be put on the importance of proper liner/interface care and the importance of lining up areas of the bony anatomy with the areas of the custom molded socket intended for those areas.

Liner care is extremely important to emphasize to prevent the chances of developing a rash or worse, an infection. If the liner is thermoplastic elastomer or silicone, the liner should be removed at the end of the day, washed with soap and water, and rinsed thoroughly to prevent residue from building up on the liner. It is vital to stress the importance of always storing the liner with the fabric facing *out*. The tackiness of the liner plays an important role in the suspension of the prosthesis on the residuum and when left facing out in an inside-out manner, particles within the air will cling to the tacky side of the liner. For example, animal hair can become embedded in the skin creating folliculitis. It is recommended that once to twice weekly, the inside of the liner be sprayed with diluted rubbing alcohol and allowed to air dry in the fabric-side out manner to prevent the growth of bacteria.

Donning liners require that special attention be paid to technique. It is imperative that there is contact between the distal end of the residuum and the most distal aspect of the liner. This requires the liner to be turned completely inside out. If there is no contact of the distal-most point of the residuum with the liner, the liner will act as a suction cup on the end of the residuum, creating a "hickey" and the potential for blistering. There should be no air pockets within the liner!

When donning socks, the patient should be educated on the importance of a smooth sock surface. Wrinkles will create areas of pressure, areas of pressure will create skin breakdown, and wounds keep a patient out of the sock while healing. The posterior aspect of the limb is an area often forgotten when trying to account for wrinkles, so be sure to provide the patient with a bendable mirror to inspect the back of the limb to ensure that wrinkles are not present in socks. Also, socks are often donned with full tension on the socks as patients attempt to remove wrinkles by pulling the socks tightly on the limb. The wearer should be encouraged to lay the sock on the residuum without pulling the sock into place and to remove wrinkles by running pads of fingers in a distal to proximal direction to work wrinkles out.

When it comes to donning the socket in the right orientation to the limb, the practitioner should demonstrate donning with respect to bony prominences and bony landmarks when training. The fibular head in the transtibial amputation is an area the prosthetist should be cautious to allow clearance due to the bony protrusion of the fibular head. If the wearer dons the prosthesis in slight internal or external rotation, the area that was intended for the fibular head will no longer line up with the fibular head, therefore creating redness and skin wearing/breakdown. This also reigns true for the use of sock ply. In donning, if the wearer has too many or too few socks on, the fibular head will not seat itself into the relief, which is the area of the socket molded in a concave design to allow space for a bony prominence.

The transtibial wearer must be cautious about bony landmarks, whereas the transfemoral wearer has little to worry about when it comes to bony protrusions; but there is challenge in donning the transfemoral socket. The Ischial Containment (IC) socket requires that the ischial tuberosity of the patient remain seated on the ischial strut in the posterior/medial corner of the diamond shaped socket. That said, many wearers will attempt to move the ischial strut in the lateral direction by turning the socket in a counter-clockwise direction thus donning the limb in an internally rotated position. When the prosthetist is aligning the transfemoral socket, the knee is placed in slight external rotation (2°–3°) in addition to the slight external rotation of the foot (1°–2°); when looking down at the prosthesis, the new wearer will want to turn the foot to face directly forward as most wearers are not aware that natural external rotation is present in all humans. When the patient dons the prosthesis with this internal rotation, the ischium is no longer on the strut and the normal rollover of the foot and clearance of the toe become more challenging.

Gait Training

Although all new prosthetic wearers are anxious to get started on walking, basic pre-gait activities are important components for setting in place good technique, strength and discipline. Pre-gait activities focus on weight shifting onto the prosthesis, balance, and breaking down the gait cycle to ensure that the individual does not create bad habits when learning to ambulate.

Weight shift exercises create confidence and are the building blocks of learning prosthetic trust. Prosthetic trust is evident in the phase at midstance when standing on the prosthesis, while being in midswing with the sound limb; it is at this time that the wearer is balancing on a prosthetic limb, which is not "part of their body," when the center of mass is as far from the ground as it gets throughout the cycle. Progression of the exercise is recommended when the prosthetic wearer is able to tap up with control, with no hand held assist, and with control of the weight shift. Tap ups are a common exercise and can be used for assessment purposes as well as training and can be progressed as the patient improves. Tap ups require a step or box starting with a height of 1 to 2 inches and progressing to a higher step. The patient is instructed to hold onto parallel bars with both hands and slowly and with control, shift the weight onto the prosthetic side as they lift their non-affected, sound limb to tap up onto the box, and then return the sound limb to the floor. This exercise appears easy, but the challenge is in the control of the weight shift onto the prosthesis.

Breaking down the gait cycle can be effective in teaching the patient the placement of the prosthesis at all times in the gait cycle as well as giving the patient and the provider the opportunity to discuss when gait deviations will occur. A common exercise to start with is the heel-to-toe rollover in the parallel bars of the prosthetic limb. This exercise is especially effective when working with the transfemoral population as it gives the new wearer a chance to learn the mechanics of the knee to learn what triggers the knee to bend and when in the cycle it will bend. This exercise simply requires the patient to place the prosthetic foot at a "comfortable" distance in front to advance the limb as if taking a step and to encourage heel-to-toe rollover. A comfortable distance to the new learner may be a longer step than the opposite limb, so it is important to take this opportunity to guide the patient toward a more normal and equal step length to that which the sound limb will take.

6

Definitive or "Permanent" Prosthesis

John Fox

A prosthesis is a replacement for a missing limb or part of a limb, which meets accepted standards for comfort, fit, alignment, function, appearance, and durability. Ongoing tissue atrophy, weight, physical changes, etc., that require further prosthetic changes undermine the custom of classifying a transtibial (TT) prosthesis as permanent or definitive.

There are several other TT prosthetic designs but those listed below are the most commonly used today. The type of prosthesis is determined by a multitude of factors, including, but not limited to, activity level, residual limb length and shape, diagnosis, and prognosis.

BELOW-KNEE PROSTHESIS: PATELLAR TENDON BEARING (PTB)

The patellar tendon bearing (PTB) socket is the basis for almost all below-knee (BK) prostheses. It provides some weight-bearing support in the area of the patellar tendon, popliteal fossa, and medial tibial flare. There are many variants of the PTB prosthesis (Figure 6.1).

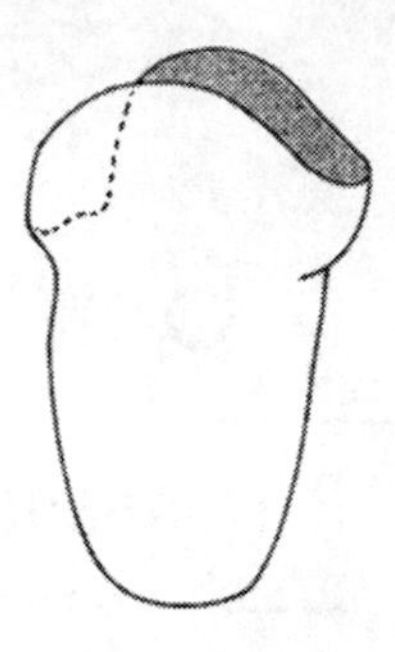

Figure 6.1 Patellar tendon bearing (PTB) socket.

Supracondylar

In this case, the PTB socket is extended proximally above the knee. This socket design is primarily used on short residual limbs for better control and a knee that has lateral/medial knee instability. The socket can be designed to be donned by pushing downward into the socket past the narrower proximal portion and "popping in." It can also utilize a removable medial wedge that is removed for donning and replaced after the prosthesis is on. Both these designs provide the necessary suspension to keep the prosthesis on (Figure 6.2).

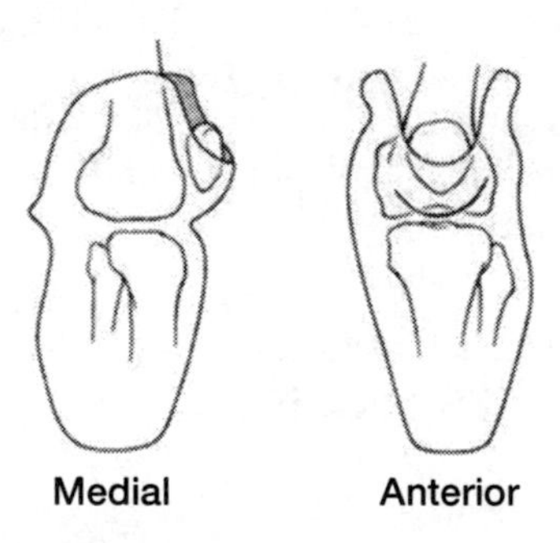

Figure 6.2 PTB-SC socket.

Supracondylar/Suprapatellar

This type of suspension has the same characteristics as the supracondylar type, reduces hyperextension of the knee, and provides more weight-bearing surface. Enclosing the patella restricts some motion and it can be difficult to fit muscular or obese thighs (Figure 6.3).

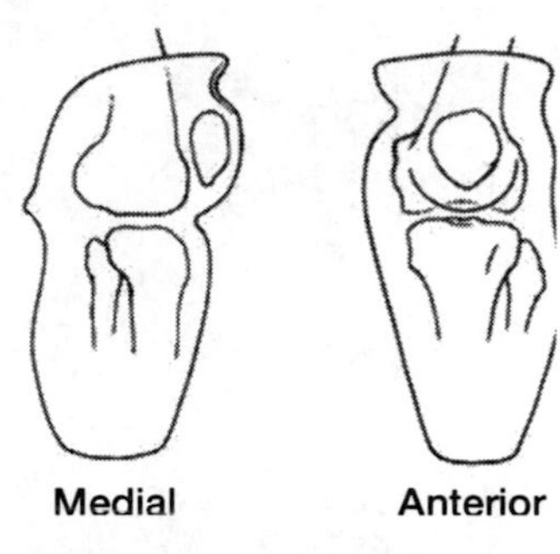

Figure 6.3 PTB-SCSP socket.

Total Surface Bearing (TSB)

This socket distributes weight-bearing over the entire residual limb. The increased surface area reduces the amount of pressure uniformly.

Joint and Corset

This system is rarely used today and only in special circumstances such as for a residual limb that cannot tolerate any weight-bearing on the distal end. It provides better control for a knee that has lateral/medial or hyperextension instability (Figure 6.4).

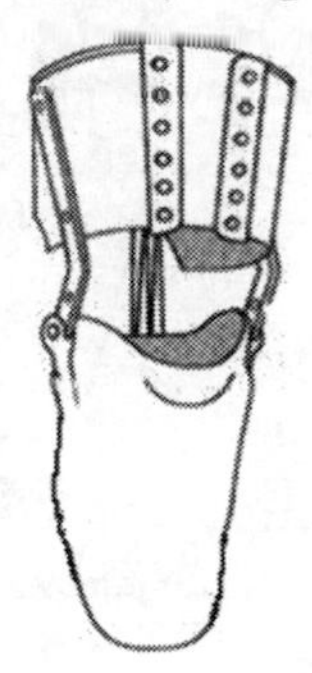

Figure 6.4 PTB socket with joints and corset.

SUPPLEMENTAL SUSPENSION SYSTEMS TO KEEP THE PROSTHESIS ON THE RESIDUAL LIMB

Waist Belt, Fork Strap, and Cuff

Although not generally used today, these suspension methods can be used for the patient who has skin reactions to silicone and/or other chemically fabricated liners (Figure 6.5).

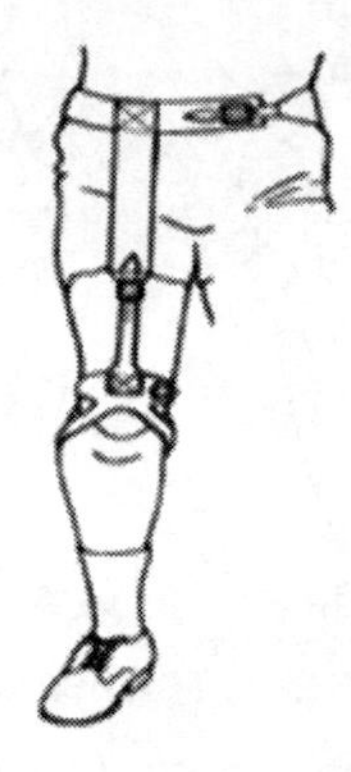

Figure 6.5 Waist belt, fork strap and PTB cuff used for suspension.

Supracondylar Wedge

This wedge locks the prosthesis by applying pressure to the medial condyle. The wedge may be removable or flexible enough to allow the condyle to push into the socket (Figure 6.6).

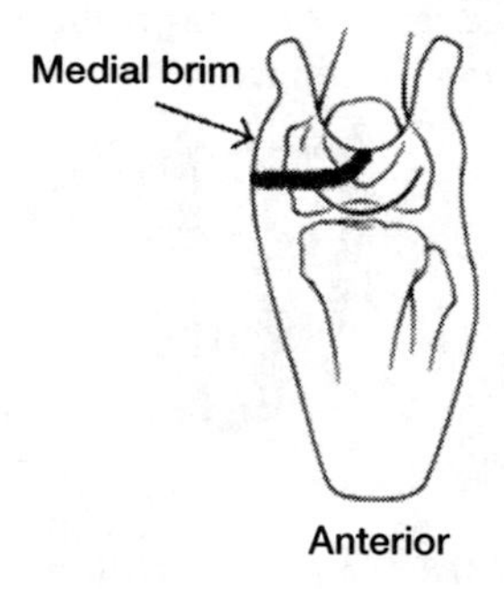

Figure 6.6 PTB-SC with removable wedge socket.

Silicone Locking Liner

This is the most commonly used suspension today. A silicone liner is rolled onto the patient's residual limb and a vacuum seal is created. The distal end of the liner has a protruding pin that enters the lock, which is incorporated into the distal end of the prosthetic socket. This suspension can also use a lanyard or strap in place of the pin lock. The lanyard is useful for those patients who have difficulty aligning the pin to the lock when donning a prosthesis (Figure 6.7).

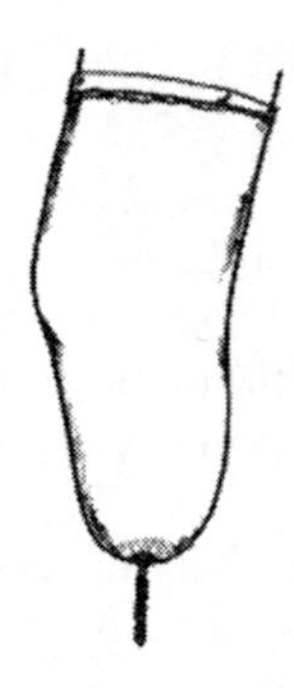

Figure 6.7 Silicone liner with locking pin.

Silicone Suction Liner

This suspension uses a liner exactly as the locking liner without the pin. The liner is rolled onto the patient in the same manner and then with the liner on, the residual limb is inserted into the suction socket, which has a one-way air expulsion valve. An outer suspension sleeve is placed on the outside of the socket and then rolled proximally until it makes contact with the skin thus creating a sealed environment. The patient will expel the remaining air from the prosthesis upon standing and thus create a suction suspension (Figure 6.8).

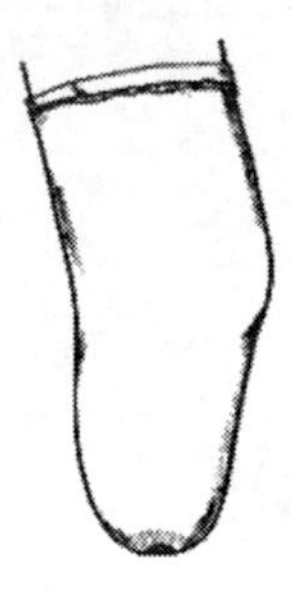

Figure 6.8 Silicone liner used for suction socket.

FEET AND COMPONENTRY

1. **Non-Articulating (Flexible Keel):** Non-articulating feet are rigid and cannot bend. The heel compresses at weight-bearing, and the flexible forefoot allows rollover. The solid ankle cushion heel (SACH) foot is an example of a non-articulating foot.

2. **Single-Axis:** Single-axis feet have joints that articulate up and down in the sagittal plane and aid in knee stability.
3. **Multi-Axis:** Multi-axis feet conform to more uneven surfaces and provide motion in all planes.
4. **Dynamic Response:** Dynamic response feet store and release energy. There are a multitude of these feet available, for various activities including sports. They are often referred to as carbon fiber feet.
5. **Microprocessor Feet:** Microprocessor feet monitor and control the functions and capabilities of the foot electronically as in the microprocessor knees.

There are a multitude of prosthetic feet available commercially, and different factors influence their choice. For example: A TT prosthesis, with a long residual limb length 8–10" or more may not accommodate a prosthetic foot that has a tall build height. Thus a different foot will need to be chosen that can fit within the build height restrictions.

Additional components, such as rotators and shock absorbers, can be used as long as the build height allows.

7

Lower Extremity Prosthetic Componentry

Shaun O'Brien

In this chapter, we will break down lower extremity componentry into three basic categories: prosthetic feet and knees. There have been many innovations over the years, some so successful that they remain relevant after decades while others had short shelf lives and have been replaced by improved technologies. In what follows, we will address the prosthetic devices currently in use by clinicians and patients. We will attempt to explore the functional characteristics and prescription criteria of each, starting with the most fundamental devices and progress to the latest technologies. These components act as the primary interface between the amputee and the ground, dispersing forces, creating or alleviating socket pressures, providing stability, and permitting a variety of daily activities.

FEET

SACH

The solid ankle cushion heel (SACH) foot is the most basic prosthetic foot still used in practice today. It is comprised of a willow wood keel extending from the ankle to the forefoot [1]. The exterior is made up of blown, baked polyurethane foam with a canvas plantar belting. The heel is the most dynamic component of the unit and varies in its level of hardness depending on the compression desired in the early stance phase of the gait cycle [2]. This compression allows for the simulation of the sound foot's plantar flexion.

The SACH foot was developed in the 1950s and has fallen behind its competitors in the ability to effectively replicate human gait. It remains a low cost option for the third world [2] and offers a durable option for both children and adults who prefer exoskeletal prostheses for water, industrial, or mechanical activities. These examples excluded, this foot has proven too stiff to be considered a foot of choice for the average to active lower extremity amputee. A study was conducted by the Veterans Administration, with 179 amputees; "excessive foot stiffness" was noted as the fundamental concern with performance [2].

Single Axis

The single axis foot technology was popularized by JE Hanger, the first amputee of the American Civil War [2]. The foot is composed of an ankle unit, usually comprised of steel or titanium, two rubber bumpers of different densities depending on the weight and needs of the patient, and a foot component which varies from manufacturer to manufacturer. Most companies create a rubber or polyurethane foam foot, with an inner core of Delrin®, carbon, or belting providing additional dynamic properties to the ankle function.

The relevance of this technology remains true today. It is a basic construction and design, but is unrivaled in its ability to aid the amputee in plantar flexing to achieve foot flat, in a short duration. This is a benefit to the new above-knee (AK) amputee who is undergoing both physical therapy and gait training. The result of increased contact with the ground allows for greater stability and subsequently greater control of the prosthetic knee joint [3]. Another indication for use of the single axis foot is the elderly below-knee (BK) amputee who desires a light-weight foot and perceived ankle motion. This individual would be a limited ambulator.

Flexible Keel (Energy Storing) Foot

The most common flexible keel foot in production today is the Seattle light foot. This foot was developed by Prosthetic Research Study and Boeing aircraft in 1981, with the goal of providing the amputee the ability to run and engage in sporting activities [4]. At its core is a Delrin keel which acts like a leaf spring, loading and unloading during weight bearing. This is the first foot to utilize this technology, which has become widely known in the industry as energy storing.

The product has evolved and the manufacturer now offers a carbon based version, with even greater advantages to the amputee. Both of these keels are embedded in a natural polyurethane molded casing.

This technology has provided a foundation that has propelled the industry forward in thinking about what role a prosthesis can play in an individual's life. The amputee could begin to think about their future in terms of actions outside activities of daily living (ADL). It would become the challenge of the prosthetist and the engineering community to keep up with the needs of the patient. As with most new technologies, the energy storing foot concept had just been developed, an evolution that was to take many new forms over future decades.

What keeps the Seattle light foot relevant today is its basic function and low cost. It can be successfully utilized with a multi-axial ankle to provide increased motion and activity. Indications for this technology would be the average to moderately active patient looking for a less expensive solution to their needs.

Energy Storing Carbon Feet

The Seattle light foot opened the door to the most influential advancement of prosthetic technology to date, the energy storing carbon foot. This technology was created by the collaboration of a plastics engineer and a young research prosthetist. The company they started, Flex Foot Inc., in 1984 spawned a new generation of thinking and a product, or its variations, which is still used by some 90% of paralympic athletes [5].

The carbon foot maintains the energy storing characteristics of the Seattle light foot, but with an improved design. The product was created with a patented J shape that allowed the foot to store energy as the patient loaded weight from heel strike to midstance, and release that energy from midstance to toe off. This foot focuses on the dynamic properties of carbon graphite composite from the socket or connection point (pylon) to the ground. Each foot is designed to the specific patient's needs, compiled from data such as weight and activity level. The carbon is manufactured in an ultra-high pressure, high temperature molding process to ensure a maximum strength-to-weight ratio and limit chances of failures. To further limit any interference of the dynamic properties of the material itself, the carbon foot is incased in a removable foot shell, not embedded in an injected molded casing. Most feet on the market today have a base of carbon composite technology, and a variation of the J shape. The author does not feel that the impact of the flex foot on the industry of prosthetics can be overstated [4].

Powered and Computerized Feet

The latest advancement in prosthetic feet comes in the form of computerized powered dorsiflexion and plantarflexion. Similar technology has been utilized in knees for well over a decade; only recently have engineers found a way to apply this computer aided technology with active plantarflexion to mimic the gastroc and soleus muscle's natural ability to propel the human foot forward at toe off. The main inhibiting factor to this advancement was twofold: one, the ability to create mechanical power, and two, how to store and release that power in an easy-to-attach and light-weight battery.

An innovation of this magnitude took significant research, development, and funding. In the world of computer aided knees, Otto Bock took on this burden of advancement. However, in the realm of the prosthetic foot, it was Ossur who took the risk and worked with insurance companies to ensure that this technology had a chance to help the lives of patients throughout the world.

The first version of this foot was deemed the "Proprio" and was released in 2007. At its core lies the basic low profile flex foot. The carbon energy storing foot's dynamic properties remain unmatched. Incorporated into the unit is an ankle module that adjusts, via accelerometers and angle sensors, to various terrains. This allows the foot to dorsiflex or plantarflex to the precise angle of incline/decline. Hills and slopes have always presented a challenge to the average BK amputee. Even a fluid ambulator would be required to change their gait pattern and adopt either one of the two methods: side step or toe/heel walk. This presents the unilateral amputee with an unstable situation and the bilateral an insurmountable task for all but the most agile and balanced patients.

The next generation of this technology was released in 2011, and was named the "iWalk." This was a collaboration of MIT research and government funding. As the result of wartime casualties, the U.S. government invested tens of millions of dollars in developing new technologies for wounded warriors coming home stateside [6]. The goal was to improve the lives of these individuals, allowing them the opportunity to resume their lives, pursue career opportunities in both the public and the private sector, as well as, in some cases return to active duty.

The iWalk used computer aided technology and active dorsiflexion, as well. The major improvement was its ability to provide power for the first time in the evolution of the artificial foot. It replicated the muscle function of the gastroc and soleus providing a push at the end of the gait cycle. This provides the amputee the ability to provide equal advancement of both extremities without relying on the sound limb for a larger percentage of the energy output. At its core lies the carbon energy storing foot, which remains a solid basic source of support and flexibility. The millions of dollars and hours of manpower devoted to technologies, such as these, advance the field of prosthetics and turn the path in a new direction, thereby providing a future generation of engineers and prosthetists the challenge of getting even closer to replicating the natural function of a lost limb.

The drawback of this technology is the weight of the battery and ankle module. In most cases, it doubles the load of the artificial limb. As a result, there tends to be increased issues with suspension. Prosthetists, in general, prefer suction or vacuum as the method of attachment for this technology. Also, the patient needs to be cognitively able to handle maintenance and charging. There are no specific patient indications for this technology; however, both of these companies have released the products solely for unilateral amputees. As advancements are made, there can be applications for both bilateral BK and AK amputees. This technology is still progressing, but its implications for future applications are endless.

Rotation/Shock/Multi-Axis Units

While the energy storing carbon foot remains the benchmark of design, at this point in time, innovation continues to be applied to this basic design. Many manufacturers attempt to incorporate the additional features of rotation, shock, and multi-axial motion into the design of the foot. Some are successful and for others it is merely an added feature or weight, not significantly improving the patient's life or adding functionality to an activity. For the simplicity of this chapter, we will explain these various designs as additional components.

Rotation can be achieved through the use of springs or compression of rods. It is an effective solution for a patient experiencing sheer forces as the result of rotational friction [7]. More than that, it is useful for active amputees who wish to engage in activities requiring rotation, such as golf and swinging a baseball bat. The argument for a short residual limb requiring the use of rotators to reduce friction over a reduced surface area, has been made over the years. In practice, the weight does not outweigh the benefit of this statement. Most short residual limb patients will request a lighter prosthesis over rotational function. Weight and suspension are greater concerns, the shorter the limb.

Next we will discuss shock absorption. This has been achieved in several ways by using the compression of springs, air, or oil. In many manufacturing designs, the rotation is built into the unit as well, providing additional function to the patient. Shock units provide the amputee the ability to sustain a higher impact from ground reaction forces resulting from such activities as jumping. One sport where the weight is secondary to function, in terms of this unit, is basketball. An active amputee who chooses to play such a sport will want to work with his prosthetist and select a shock absorber that is appropriate.

Lastly, let us discuss multi-axial units. In most cases, this technology is relatively light and easily incorporated. Some manufacturers incorporate it into the foot unit itself as an interface between the carbon components. When this is done, the benefit is added motion in the coronal plane. Unfortunately, it comes at the expense of limiting some of the dynamic properties inherent in the carbon itself. The patients often describe experiencing a dead spot in midstance. A multi-axial unit attached above the foot component itself will increase the motion in both the coronal and the sagittal plane. This motion can be beneficial to less dynamic feet or for a patient who spends much time on uneven ground, such as outdoors. This technology has many uses for both the active amputee and the average ambulatory who have challenges requiring additional consideration.

KNEES

Single Axis

This is the most fundamental knee available today. It is comprised of one axis point, a bolt with mechanical friction being the only adjustment available [8]. Increasing this friction allows the prosthetist to limit heel rise and extension. Knee stability is achieved through the proper placement of the knee axis in relation to the Trochanter Knee Ankle (TKA) line. Knee stability depends on the relation of the TKA line the center of the knee axis. The more posterior this line is to the knee axis the more the knee has a tendency to flex. Moving the TKA line more anteriorly causes the knee to be more stable but may increase the difficulty of flexing the knee. This placement is determined by the preference of the patient, the physical evaluation of the physical rehabilitation team, and the experience of the prosthetist. This knee is rarely used in modern practice, due to its simplistic design and lack of features. It will, at times, be used by amputees who request a light-weight exoskeletal prosthesis.

Manual Locking

This feature can be added to a variety of knees but is most commonly applied to the single axis modular unit. The lack of swing feature limits the need for a more complex, heavy, or cost prohibitive design. The basic single axis knee is modified to incorporate a locking mechanism attached to a mechanical release located proximally on the AK socket. For the geriatric patient who lacks the strength to maintain a standing position unassisted, but has the potential for increased mobility or desires a prosthesis for simple ADL such as transfers, standing and washing dishes, etc., this knee is an appropriate option. The patient still needs to meet the minimum requirements for a prosthesis, but for those with limited potential this is the right choice. As the amputee progresses in their functional capabilities, the individual can advance to a knee that allows for flexion. A locking knee, if used for prolonged ambulation, can cause improper gait habits and lumbar pain.

Weight Activated Locking

This is the next step in knee technology currently in use today. This knee has two axes of rotation [8] and a mechanical brake, made up of a spring coil that expands when the patient's weight is applied. The original design, still in production, has constant friction as a swing phase monitor. Current designs come with pneumatic and even hydraulic controls. Often you will see extension assists offered with this technology and other mechanical knees available. This knee provides a heightened sense of security and is appropriate for the elderly amputee population.

Polycentric Knees

This knee provides additional stability to the amputee through the engineering achievements of multiple axes of rotation. It is often called a four-bar knee, due to the fact that its original design was comprised of four bars and four axes of rotation. Additional axes of rotation and additional bars (up to six) have been added to this design, all in an attempt to move the mechanical center of rotation behind the perceived axis of rotation. The advantage to the amputee is knee stability without the need for a mechanical lock; thus the patient can quickly progress from full extension into swing phase and knee flexion. For the average amputee with good strength, range of motion, and stability, this provides a good option for the preparatory prosthesis. It can be used to teach proper gait technique, build strength and balance, and assess functional potential. Additional swing phase features, such as pneumatic and hydraulic controls, are also available for this design.

Hydraulic

The hydraulic knee most commonly known in the field of prosthetics is the Mauch SNS (swing and stance) control. While many of the mechanical knees mentioned above are available today in hydraulic or pneumatic swing phase controls, in its time, the Mauch knee was the first of its kind [9]. It offered a hydraulic stance phase feature that allowed the amputee adjustable stability and provided knee flexion throughout the stance phase. The result was a more natural gait and an increase in activity for the patient. This knee allowed patients more control over their prosthesis and improved the quality of life for many. A drawback of this design was that it was for individuals who had not only good strength, range of motion, and balance, but who also had developed effective prosthetic gait habits previously. While the knee provides hydraulic swing and stance controls, it still maintains one axis of rotation. Thus, the amputee must ultimately control the knee during the stance phase. They can allow the resistance to provide some natural knee flexion in midstance but must be firing their hip extensors to remain standing. Again, the SNS unit is a very effective and still a relevant design for the average to active amputee.

MPK – Microprocessor Controlled Knee

The first company to come out with this design was Otto Bock, in 1997 [10]. The knee was called the C-Leg and was the most technologically advanced device of its time. How many feet have been built off the basic design of the carbon flex foot? The C-Leg was a digitally controlled version of the basic SNS unit. What were the significant advantages of computer aided technology adjusting the various values controlling both stance and swing phase of gait?

Stability

Previously the Mauch knee, for example, had one setting and if the amputee wanted to run or increase their cadence they needed to have multiple prostheses or go to the prosthetist to have their knee adjusted. Some may have been given the settings to adjust it themselves, but for liability rationale, this is not common practice. The microprocessor allowed the prosthetist to take multiple settings. Two settings were provided in the first version, with the ability of the amputee to adjust between them at will; more importantly than this was the knee's stumble recovery mode. This allowed the patient to ride the knee down ramps and stairs, as well as, have confidence in the knee if they took a misstep. The knee had sensors that the microprocessor monitored and through information from the sensors about joint angles the microprocessor controlled the rate at which hydraulic valves opened and closed for the most appropriate gait patterns and stability. If the patient took a misstep and the weight remained behind the toe the knee began to tighten up behind the toe, resistance to knee flexion increased to keep the amputee from falling. This technology, first made available for the average to active amputee, began to show benefits for the geriatric or less confident ambulator. As a result of the stumble recovery mode, a less active version of this knee became available for a larger segment of the population.

There are a variety of companies producing MPKs in today's market. Some learn and adjust to the amputee. As the amputee increases his cadence so does the knee, and the patient no longer has to self-select. Some knees are controlled by a metallic viscous fluid that changes consistencies as a charge is applied, changing the rate at which the flexes extend. This knee, in particular, is known for its fluid and natural cycle. Certain manufacturers produce waterproof versions with less pronounced safety features and a quicker response time for more active individuals. Another brand just released its latest model in 2011 (the X2 from Otto Bock), which allows individuals the freedom to kick a ball and ascend the stairs by utilizing the resistance in the knee and advancements in both sensor and gyroscope technology. MPKs are an appropriate choice for any level of amputee so long as they show the potential for independent/unassisted ambulation and full time prosthetic wear. Contraindications for this device are weight, maintenance, cognitive ability, and cost.

Power Knee

In the previous section, we mentioned an MPK, the X2, that was released in 2011. This knee allows the amputee to ascend stairs with its advancements in sensor and gyroscopic technology. This is a major accomplishment for the industry and the lives of the amputees affected. The knee is a relatively light-weight product due to its lack of powered extension. There is no aspect of the knee that mimics the human muscle tissue or generates power. The amputee self-initiates all movements at the hip, which results in an overall increase of more than 200% in energy expenditure. Ossur's Power Knee was the first knee to attempt to add this feature; it was released in 2006 [11]. The knee provided powered extension. The amputee wore a sensor on the sound limb and the computer aided artificial knee mimicked this movement on the contralateral side. An amputee could really ascend a graded incline or stairs. Power was provided at the knee, thus reducing the need for the amputee to generate all forces with his remaining residual limb. As with any new advancement, there are drawbacks and counter indications. Power knees represent a technology, that with further refinements, has much to offer amputees. One of its current drawbacks is the noise that it produces. With its current design, the indications for this technology would be the younger, active amputee. This is exciting technology and its applications are limitless.

REFERENCES

1. Bakalim G. *Experiences With the PTB Prosthesis, Selected Articles from Artificial Limbs*. Huntington, NY, Krieger Publishing, pp. 363–371.
2. Ayyappa, E. *Prosthetic Desk Reference*. Long Beach, CA: Department of Veterans Affairs; 1997, pp. 37–43.
3. Hornbeak S, Staats, T. *Below Knee Reader I*. Dominguez Hills, CA.
4. *Chapter – Lower Limb Components*. State University; 2004, pp. 1–7.
5. Micheal J. *Clinical Prosthetics and Orthotics*. Vol. 11, No. 3. The American Academy of Orthotists and Prosthetists; 1987, pp. 154–168.
6. Inventor of the Week, January 2007: Van Phillips; Lemelson-MIT program; http://web.mit.edu/invent/iow/phillips.html; Retrieved 2008-07-02.
7. The iWalk Story; http://www.iwalkpro.com/iwalkstory.html; Retrieved March 2012.
8. Tindall GA, Nitschke RO. The ROL rotator. *Ortho Prosth*. 1979;33(1):11–15.
9. Muilenburg AL, Wilson BA Jr. A *Manual for Above-Knee Amputees*. Huston, TX; 1984, pp. 13–17.
10. Wilson AB. Hydraulics and trans-femoral prosthetics. *Clin Prosth Ortho*. 1983;7(4):3–4.
11. Martin CW. *Otto Bock C-Leg: A Review of its Effectiveness*. WCB Evidence Based Group; 2003.

8

Partial Foot Amputation

Joseph Webster

Partial foot amputations present a unique set of challenges from both a surgical and a rehabilitation perspective. Although the functional outcomes of partial foot amputations compared to higher levels of amputation remain unclear, this level of amputation is being utilized more commonly in persons with vascular disease as well as those with traumatic limb injuries. While retention of a portion of the foot has the potential to offer some individuals a functional and cosmetic advantage, this level of amputation has traditionally been associated with an increased likelihood of skin breakdown and the need for surgical revision [1]. There are various prosthetic and/or orthotic options available for the person with a partial foot amputation depending on the amputation level and the person's functional goals. Advances in technology and product designs have resulted in the availability of newer types of partial foot prostheses, orthoses, and shoe wear [1]. While a diversity of orthotic and prosthetic devices have been developed for use by persons with partial foot amputations, their comparative functional characteristics and outcomes have not been well quantified. In addition, while prior studies have shown that partial foot amputations affect the biomechanics of gait, there is limited research examining the influence of prosthetic and orthotic intervention on these gait variables [2,3].

This chapter will cover the epidemiology of partial foot amputations as well as surgical approaches, advantages, disadvantages, and prosthetic/orthotic management for each commonly seen level of partial foot amputation. Table 8.1 provides the overall classification of partial foot amputations and Figure 8.1 demonstrates the various levels of partial foot amputations.

OVERALL CLASSIFICATION

Table 8.1 Overall Classification of Partial Foot Amputations

Forefoot amputations
Toe
Ray
Midfoot amputations
Transmetatarsal
Lisfranc (tarsal–metatarsal disarticulation)
Hindfoot amputations
Chopart (transtarsal by sparing calcaneus and talus)
Boyd and Pirogoff (transtarsal with partial calcanectomy)

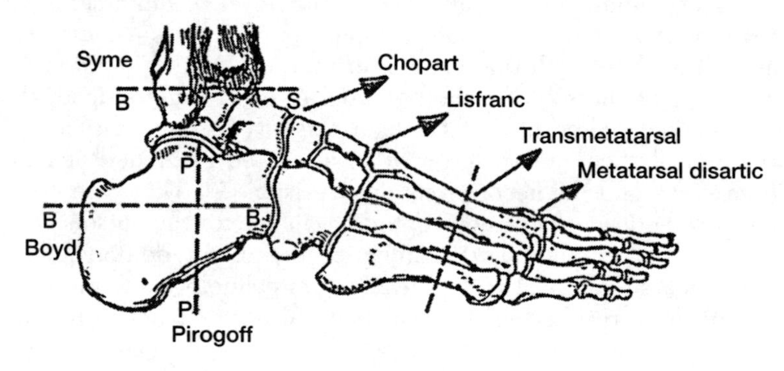

Figure 8.1 Levels of partial foot amputations.

Epidemiology

Toe amputations are a very common level of amputation in persons with peripheral vascular disease and diabetes. While this level of amputation is very common, its functional impact is low. More proximal partial foot amputations have historically represented a relatively smaller percentage of lower extremity amputations, but this level of amputation has increased in recent years with the increase in revascularization procedures and attempts at limb salvage. Some authors consider all partial foot amputations to be in the minor amputation category whereas others classify amputations at the transmetarsal level and more proximal as major amputations [4–14].

Toe and partial foot amputations account for approximately 42% of all dysvascular amputations [4].

Toe and partial foot amputations account for 16% of all civilian traumatic amputations [4].

The most common civilian traumas resulting in partial foot amputations are lawn mower injuries and motor vehicle accidents. Others etiologies include crush injuries with or without fractures, degloving injuries, and thermal injuries [1].

Toe and partial foot amputations account for 3.4% of all combat-related traumatic amputations in Operation Enduring Freedom/ Operation Iraqi Freedom (OEF/OIF) Service members (5% of all combat-related lower extremity amputations) [5,6].

Progression to a higher level of amputation is common in patients with partial foot amputations [7,8].

37% to 40% of patients with diabetes and initial amputation at the toe or partial foot/ankle level will require an additional amputation within one year [7,8].

Male gender, race, older age, and diabetes are risk factors for partial foot amputations [9–11].

Among patients with diabetes treated in the Veterans Affairs (VA), rates of initial minor amputations (ankle disarticulation and distal) are almost double the rate of major amputations (4.5 vs. 2.4) [11].

Rates of both minor amputations (33%) and major amputations (36%) decreased over a five-year study period from 2000 to 2004 among patients with diabetes treated in the VA [11].

Over a 10-year time period, an increasing trend in the percentage of minor amputations compared to major amputations has been noted [12].

Toe Amputation

Overview

This is the most common level of amputation secondary to vascular disease and diabetes.

Surgical Considerations

The surgical procedure for toe amputations is relatively uncomplicated and low risk. The first (great) toe amputation can be a reasonable amputation choice if no proximal skin breakdown is present and vascular supply will allow for distal healing. With toe amputations, it is generally recommended to leave the base of the proximal phalanx to keep both the sesamoids and the plantar fat pad beneath the metatarsal head. Multiple toe amputations can be difficult to manage and limited function may result. Leaving a toe isolated by removing the toes on either side will increase its susceptibility to injury and skin breakdown. Removal of the second toe may result in a hallux valgus (bunion) deformity. To avoid this complication, a second ray amputation can be considered [1].

Advantages

Toe amputations are typically associated with minimal functional implications. Sparing the more proximal foot helps prevent collapse of the shoe at the end of the amputation, and promotes a more even step length.

Disadvantages

There is a significant risk of skin breakdown and a high likelihood of needing additional surgical intervention in the future, in patients with vascular disease and diabetes.

Prosthetic/Orthotic Management

No prosthesis is typically required for isolated toe amputations. A total-contact foot orthosis combined with a carbon fiber foot plate or steel shank may be required. The orthosis should distribute pressure evenly under the foot with relatively less pressure under vulnerable bony prominences such as the metatarsal heads, and relatively more pressure under the arch of the foot. A toe filler can help prevent movement of the remaining foot inside the shoe, but there is also a risk of skin breakdown with toe fillers especially if the toe filler is being used with digit 2–4 amputations.

Ray Amputation

Overview

Fifth ray resection is the most commonly performed ray amputation. Combined fourth and fifth ray resections can also result in reasonable outcomes.

Surgical Considerations

Ray amputations are longitudinal-type amputations that involve the removal of the phalangeal bones and the corresponding metatarsal bone (base of metatarsal may be spared or left in place). Ray amputations are generally more successful with the amputation of the lateral fourth or fifth rays than with the medial first or second rays. Single amputations of rays two, three, or four only moderately affect the width of the forefoot. Multiple ray amputations should be avoided because the foot becomes too narrow and nonfunctional. Multiple ray amputations are also at high risk for additional skin breakdown and further surgical intervention.

Advantages

Fifth or combined fourth and fifth ray resections can result in good functional outcomes and surgical risk is lower with this level of amputation compared to more proximal amputations. Prosthetic and/or orthotic intervention requirements are less compared to more proximal amputation levels. Individuals with forefoot amputations have the potential to continue bearing weight directly on the residual foot and have improved proprioceptive feedback if sensation remains in the foot. Toe and ray amputations also result in the least alteration of body image.

Disadvantages

Relatively high rates of recurrent skin breakdown and the potential need for additional surgical intervention arise, especially in patients with vascular disease and diabetes.

Prosthetic/Orthotic Management

A total-contact, custom-molded foot orthotic with a filler is the typical treatment option. A carbon fiber foot plate is also commonly beneficial for additional support and stability during ambulation. This typically requires the use of extra-depth shoes with a soft inner liner and wide toe box to accommodate the custom insert and foot plate. A rocker bottom sole can also be added if needed, especially in patients with associated deformity or pain in the more proximal aspect of the foot.

Transmetatarsal Amputation

Overview

Transmetatarsal amputations can be a successful amputation level and produce a highly acceptable functional and cosmetic outcome.

Surgical Considerations

Transmetatarsal amputation should be considered when two or more medial rays must be amputated. With a transmetatarsal level amputation, the forefoot is transversely amputated through the shaft of the metatarsals by sparing the proximal metatarsal/metatarsal base. The remaining portions of the metatarsals are usually beveled inferiorly and covered with a predominantly plantar skin flap. The length of the residual limb needs to be based on the remaining skin and soft tissue available for closure. This will ensure both closure without tension and placement of scar tissue away from areas of direct weight-bearing and shear forces. To absorb the shear and pressure forces generated during gait, the soft-tissue envelope must be mobile. The biomechanics of the foot are altered following transmetatarsal amputation with shortening of the lever arm of the foot. This frequently requires balancing with Achilles lengthening.

Advantages

Transmetatarsal amputations can result in a functional amputation level, which is also cosmetic in appearance. Weight-bearing for short distance ambulation without a prosthetic–orthotic device can be accomplished with this level of amputation. The transmetatarsal level of amputation generally has a decreased risk of recurrent skin breakdown compared to more distal partial foot amputations.

Disadvantages

Flattening of both the transverse and longitudinal arches commonly occurs. Barefoot walking after transmetatarsal amputation is impaired because of the loss of weight-bearing metatarsal heads and the elimination of forefoot pronation and supination during gait.

Prosthetic/Orthotic Management

The transmetatarsal level of amputation is the level at which the prosthetic/orthotic needs transition from specialized foot orthotics and shoe wear modifications to the use of more extensive prosthetic/orthotics. In the older geriatric patient who will be ambulating for short distances over mainly level surfaces, an extra-depth orthopedic shoe with a custom, total-contact insert and toe filler with a carbon fiber footplate may be adequate to meet the patient's functional needs. A rocker bottom shoe can be used to aid in rollover and to reduce forces on the remaining metatarsals and distal incision line. Individuals with transmetatarsal amputations who desire to be more active will typically benefit from the use of a more formal ankle–foot orthosis (AFO). The type of AFO used can vary depending on the patient's desired functional activities and other factors such as sensory loss in the residual limb, edema, and/or contracture. The AFO will commonly need to be a custom device with the incorporation of a custom, total-contact foot orthosis and toe filler. For those individuals who would benefit from more dynamic bracing, a prefabricated carbon fiber AFO can be used in combination with the custom, total-contact foot orthotic. In the case of an individual with severe sensory loss and/or significant deformity in the residual foot, a Charcot Restraint Orthotic Walker (CROW) or a similar system can be considered. These types of orthotic devices are much more restrictive and typically result in more difficulties with ambulation, but may be appropriate in the limited ambulator who is at high risk for skin breakdown or worsening deformity. These types of devices may be indicated following forefoot amputations as well if significant proximal deformity and/or sensory loss are present.

Tarsal–Metatarsal Disarticulation Amputation (Lisfranc)

Overview

This is a fairly uncommon level of amputation secondary to the risk of plantarflexion deformity of the foot and the risk of subsequent difficulties with weight-bearing and skin breakdown.

Surgical Considerations

This is a slightly more proximal amputation level compared to a transmetatarsal amputation. This amputation involves the removal of all of the metatarsals and disarticulation of the foot at the tarsal–metatarsal level. With this more proximal amputation and loss of the base of metatarsals, there is loss of insertion points for the tibialis anterior and other peroneal muscles. This requires even more care to be taken to balance the foot with Achilles tendon lengthening as well as possible reattachment of the tibialis anterior and peroneal muscle insertions.

Advantages

There are minimal advantages of this level of amputation compared to a transmetatarsal level amputation. It would be considered over a transmetatarsal amputation when a partial foot amputation is still the desired level of amputation, but there is not adequate soft tissue available for a transmetatarsal amputation or if there are processes such as osteomyelitis or tumor involving the proximal metatarsal bones.

Disadvantages

Shortening of the lever arm of the foot results in an increased risk of equinovarus deformity and contracture.

Prosthetic/Orthotic Management

Prosthetic/orthotic restoration typically involves similar options and considerations as described for the transmetatarsal level of amputation. The use of an extra-depth orthopedic shoe with a custom-molded insert and filler as well as steel or a carbon fiber foot plate may suffice for low level functional ambulation. This can be used with or without a rocker bottom. The potential impact of the rocker bottom on balance for the older individual at risk of falling always needs to be considered. Most individuals with the Lisfranc level of amputation will benefit from fitting with an AFO system with various options available as described for the transmetatarsal amputation level.

Transtarsal Amputation by Sparing the Calcaneus and Talus (Chopart)

Overview

This level of amputation is uncommonly performed, but it can be considered as an option for patients with traumatic foot injuries or tumors. This level of amputation is rarely indicated in the patient with vascular disease or diabetes.

Surgical Considerations

This amputation is performed at the transtarsal level by sparing the talus and calcaneus (Figure 8.2). Despite surgical attempts at muscle balancing, the main problem with this amputation level is plantarflexion and inversion deformity with contracture and subsequent skin breakdown. Tendon transfers can be considered in order to help rebalance the foot. Achilles tendon lengthening can also be used to reduce the risk and severity of deformity. Arthrodesis of the ankle and subtalar joint is sometimes recommended to prevent deformity and prevent instability at the subtalar joint.

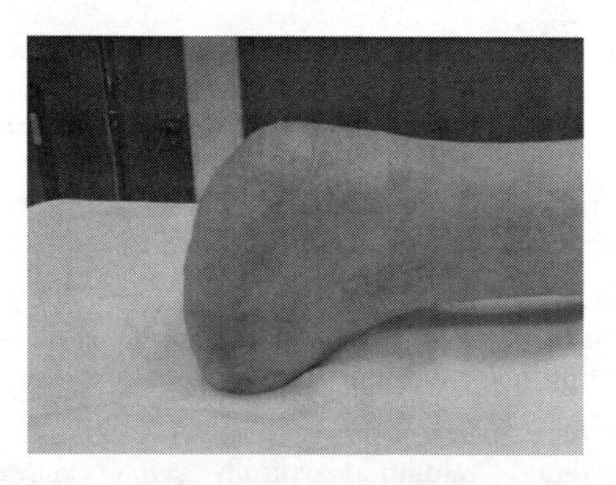

Figure 8.2 Transtarsal level (Chopart) amputation.

Advantages

Advantages include a longer lever arm compared to a transtibial level amputation, and this amputation level maintains the potential ability to perform some weight-bearing activities without the use of a prosthesis and/or orthosis.

Disadvantages

The more proximal hindfoot amputations are problematic amputations because the remaining foot is so short that there is no effective lever arm, and the remaining ankle motion is essentially nonfunctional. These levels of amputation lead to equinovarus deformities. Anterior bony prominences can develop as the heel pad migrates posteriorly. This can become painful and prone to skin breakdown.

Prosthetic/Orthotic Management

This amputation level can be difficult to fit with an adequate prosthesis and this can impact the likelihood of achieving the desired functional outcome. At the Chopart level of amputation, an AFO-style orthosis/prosthesis is usually required. The AFO needs to provide an intimate fit and extend up to the patellar tendon level to distribute the high forces that result from the torques in late stance. Lower trimlines with an active patient can result in breakdown along the crest of the tibia. Another option is the utilization of a more traditional prosthetic socket for the residual limb combined with a low profile carbon fiber prosthetic foot (Figure 8.3). With the Chopart amputation, a boot-type device can occasionally be used if there is no ankle contracture and the anterior tissues are good. Prosthetic fittings at the Chopart level can result in the need for a lift on the contralateral side to accommodate the height of the prosthesis.

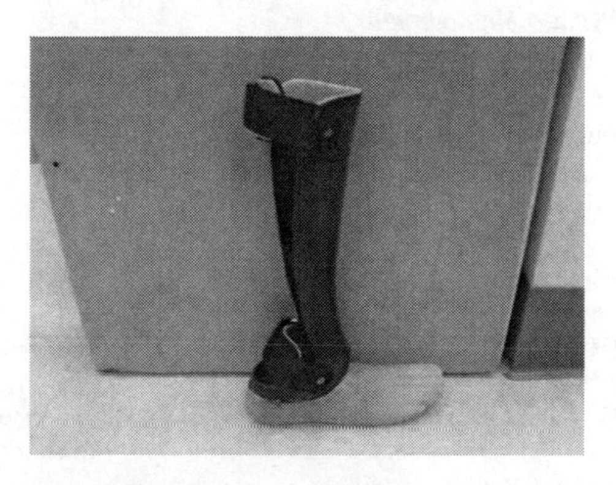

Figure 8.3 Chopart prosthetic/orthotic device.

Transtarsal Amputation With Partial Resection of the Calcaneus (Boyd/Pirogoff)

Overview

These are rarely performed levels of amputations in the adult population. Historically, these amputation levels were used more commonly in the pediatric population.

Surgical Considerations

The Boyd and Pirogoff amputations are considered partial foot amputations, but really represent variations of ankle disarticulation amputation (Symes). With the Boyd and Pirogoff amputations, only part of the calcaneus is spared and the remaining talus and calcaneus are fused to the distal tibia to lengthen the limb further and reduce limb length discrepancy. The Boyd spares the superior half of the calcaneus, whereas the Pirogoff spares the posterior portion.

Advantages

These levels of amputation can be useful in pediatric amputees when there is a desire to maintain length to accommodate future growth considerations. Because these amputations allow distal weight-bearing, this level of amputation may also be considered in situations where no prosthetic care would be available.

Disadvantages

The minimal limb shortening makes prosthetic fitting very challenging in adults. Other disadvantages are similar to those described for the Chopart level of amputation, but there is less risk of progressive deformity of the residual limb if the amputation is combined with fusion at the ankle and subtalar joint.

Prosthetic/Orthotic Management

Prosthetic/orthotic restoration typically involves similar options and considerations as described for the Chopart level of amputation. Special circumstances may need to be considered when these amputations are performed in the pediatric population.

REFERENCES

1. Bowker JH. Partial foot amputations and disarticulations: Surgical aspects. *J Prosthetics Orthotics*. 2007;19(8):62–76.
2. Dillon MP, Fatone S, Hodge MC. Biomechanics of ambulation after partial foot amputation: A systematic literature review. *J Prosthetics Orthotics*. 2007;19(8):2–61.

3. Uellendahl JE, Uellendahl EN. Summary and conclusions from the academy's eighth state-of-the-science conference, on the biomechanics of ambulation after partial foot amputation. *J Prosthetics Orthotics.* 2007;19(8):89–90.
4. Dillingham TR, Pezzin LE, MacKenzie EJ. Limb amputation and limb deficiency: Epidemiology and recent trends in the United States. *South Med J.* 2002 Aug;95(8):875–883.
5. Gailey R, McFarland LV, Cooper RA, et al. Unilateral lower-limb loss: Prosthetic device use and functional outcomes in servicemembers from Vietnam war and OIF/OEF conflicts. *J Rehabil Res Dev*. 2010;47(4):317–331.
6. Reiber GE, McFarland LV, Hubbard S, et al. Servicemembers and veterans with major traumatic limb loss from Vietnam war and OIF/OEF conflicts: Survey methods, participants, and summary findings. *J Rehabil Res Dev.* 2010;47(4):275–297.
7. Dillingham TR, Pezzin LE, Shore AD. Reamputation, mortality, and health care costs among persons with dysvascular lower-limb amputations. *Arch Phys Med Rehabil.* 2005;86(3):480–486.
8. Aulivola B, Hile CN, Hamdan AD, et al. Major lower extremity amputation: outcome of a modern series. *Arch Surg.* 2004 Apr;139(4):395–399.
9. Ephraim PL, Dillingham TR, Sector M, Pezzin LE, Mackenzie EJ. Epidemiology of limb loss and congenital limb deficiency: A review of the literature. *Arch Phys Med Rehabil.* 2003 May;84(5):747–761.
10. Norvell DC, Turner AP, Williams RM, Hakimi KN, Czerniecki JM. Defining successful mobility after lower extremity amputation for complications of peripheral vascular disease and diabetes. *J Vasc Surg*. 2011;54(2):412–419.
11. Tseng CL, Rajan M, Miller DR, Lafrance JP, Pogach L. Trends in initial lower extremity amputation rates among Veterans Health Administration health care System users from 2000 to 2004. *Diabetes Care*. 2011 May;34(5):1157–1163.
12. PACT Proclarity Cube. Amputation Briefing Book. http://vssc.med.va.gov/products.asp?PgmArea=13. Accessed 1–25–12.
13. Stone PA, Back MR, Armstrong PA, et al. Midfoot amputations expand limb salvage rates for diabetic foot infections. *Ann Vasc Surg.* 2005;19(6):805–811.
14. Nehler MR, Coll JR, Hiatt WR, et al. Functional outcome in a contemporary series of major lower extremity amputations. *J Vasc Surg.* 2003;38(1):7–14.

9

The Symes Amputation and Prosthetic Options

Terry L. Kalter

HISTORY

The Symes amputation was originally described in 1843 by James Syme, Professor of Surgery in Edinburgh, England. It is an ankle disarticulation with the removal of the malleoli and forward placement of the heel pad to protect the tibia. Syme advocated the following surgical procedures.

- The posterior tibial artery in the posterior flap must be preserved since it provides a blood supply to the heel flap. The surgical procedure has met with varied acceptance.
- The heel flap should be removed subperiosteally from the calcaneus. Due to its resiliency and natural cushioning characteristics, it provides an ideal weight-bearing medium. The heel flap should be firmly secured to the distal surface of the tibia.
- Syme said it was important to divide the tibia at the level of the dome of the ankle, parallel to the floor to achieve a good bony weight-bearing surface.

Throughout time, there have been many modifications to the Symes amputation. The most notable is that of Sarmiento in 1972, when he advocated trimming the malleoli to reduce the medial–lateral diameter of the residuum. This technique does improve the bulk and cosmesis of the prosthesis but it is still poor compared to that of a transtibial amputation. If failure of the Symes procedure were to occur, it is usually within a year of the amputation.

Indications

The most common need for a Symes amputation arises in the case of congenital deformity where growth potential should be preserved, and trauma. Its need is less where there is vascular insufficiency or infection. In these cases, a two-stage procedure is performed. Firstly, an ankle disarticulation is performed; after ensuring that no infection is present and that there is adequate blood supply, the malleoli are osteotomized and the incision is closed.

Benefits

The Symes amputation has received varied opinions on its benefits.

- The functional benefits are apparent displaying a more natural gait pattern.
- The Symes amputation gives the patient a longer lever arm for better control of the prosthesis during the gait cycle.
- There is no transection of bone, so healing time is decreased.
- For the same reason as the above, there is a decrease in pain.
- Once healed, the patient can bear weight on the end of the residuum. This has the benefit of decreasing the amount of weight needed to be borne on more proximal areas of the residual limb.
- There is no need to don a prosthesis to ambulate around the home or at the pool.
- There is an improved proprioception for foot placement.

The Downside

- A Symes amputation results in a bulbous distal end that is non-cosmetic (Figure 9.1). Women generally have greater concerns about the poor cosmesis associated with the Symes amputation.
- The limited space between the distal socket and the ground hampers the foot choice for the prosthetist.
- Successfully fitting a prosthesis is dependent on surgical expertise to minimize bony prominences and excess redundant tissue.

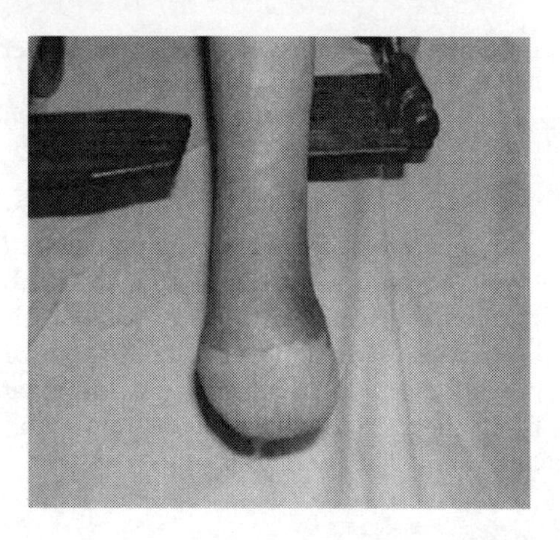

Figure 9.1 Result of a Symes amputation.

THE PRESCRIPTION

Socket Design

There are four basic types of sockets: the older leather-laced model within a metal casing or frame which is rarely used today, the plastic push-fit prosthesis with a removable expandable polyurethane foam liner (Figure 9.2), the air cushion socket (also referred to as an expandable walled socket) (Figure 9.3), and the laminated plastic socket with a removable medial door, which allows the limb to slide into place after which the window is secured with straps. The plastic push-fit prosthesis with an expandable polyurethane foam liner and the air cushion socket incorporating a flexible silicone bladder are the most cosmetically acceptable. The air cushion socket is fabricated utilizing a three-stage lamination and is a very difficult technical process. All Symes sockets usually extend to just below the patella. It may incorporate a patellar tendon bearing (PTB) design. Another socket design that is sometimes used is the Canadian Symes. It has an opening in the posterior for ease in donning. This design is not the one of choice because the posterior of the prosthesis is where the highest stress is located. The Symes prosthesis is a challenging prosthesis to fabricate due to the unique aspects of this amputation (Figure 9.4).

Suspension

The Symes prosthesis is usually self-suspending. Suspension is achieved by applying anatomically contoured medial–lateral pressure proximal to the malleoli. A supracondylar suspension strap may be used if necessary.

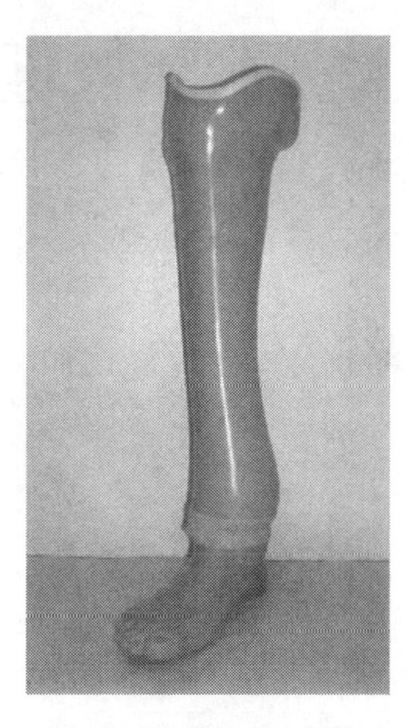

Figure 9.2 Symes prosthesis with a removable soft insert.

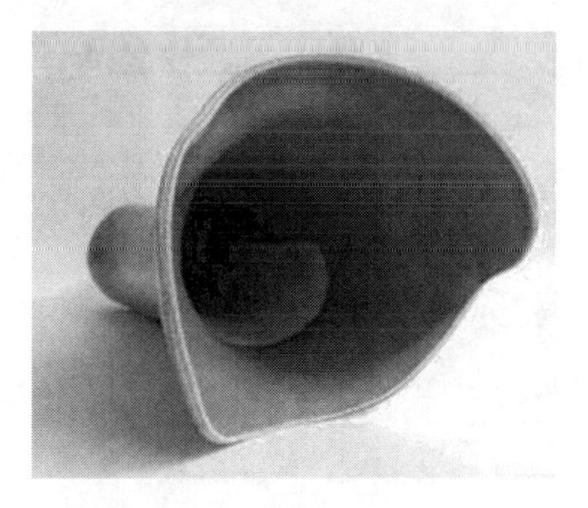

Figure 9.3 Expandable walled Symes prosthesis.

Feet

There are three main types of prosthetic feet: the rigid Pirogoff foot (Figure 9.5), usually with a wooden keel (as with the Kingsley Symes Sach foot; Figure 9.6), the flexible foot with either a delrin or carbon-fiber

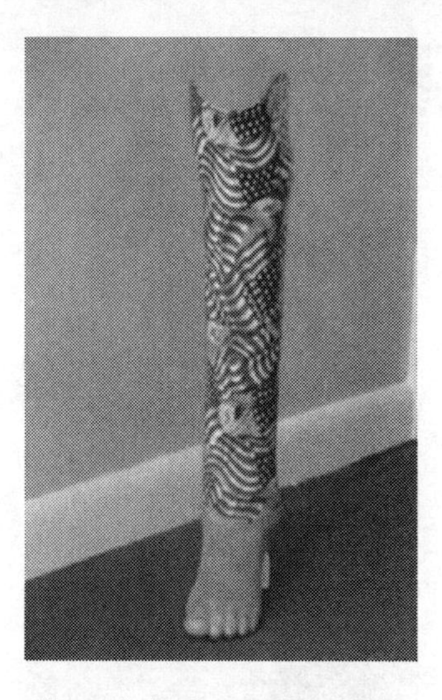

Figure 9.4 Symes prosthesis.

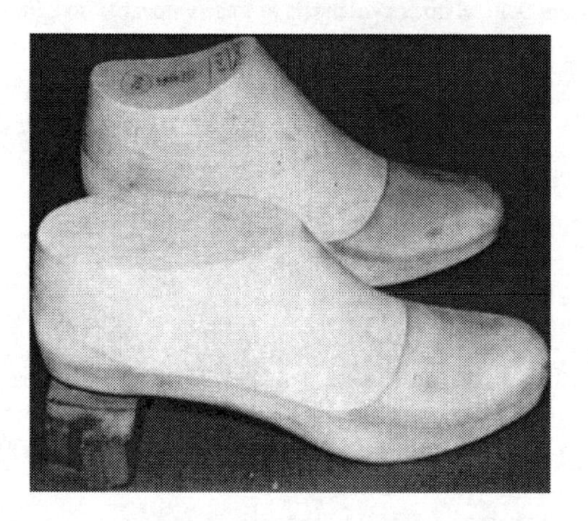

Figure 9.5 Pirogoff foot.

keel (for example, the Seattle foot and Quantum Symes foot), and the energy-storing foot, which has carbon-fiber plates inside a footshell (Figures 9.7–9.10). The rigid Pirogoff foot with its wooden keel still has the advantage over the more modern flexible dynamic response feet with the ability to accommodate a longer stump by sinking the socket into the wooden keel. The flexible Delrin® or carbon fiber feet give a

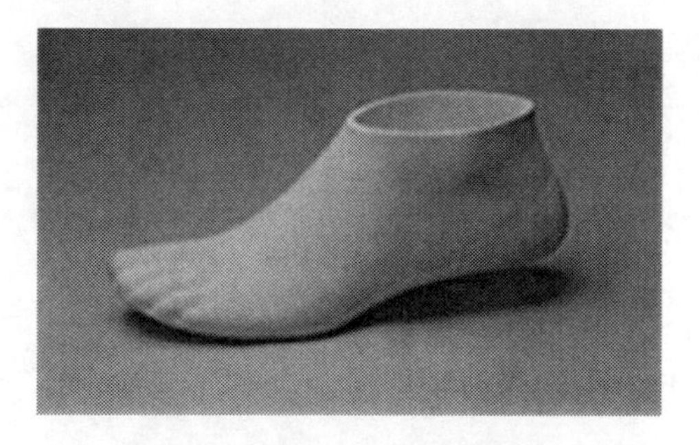

Figure 9.6 Kingsley Symes foot.

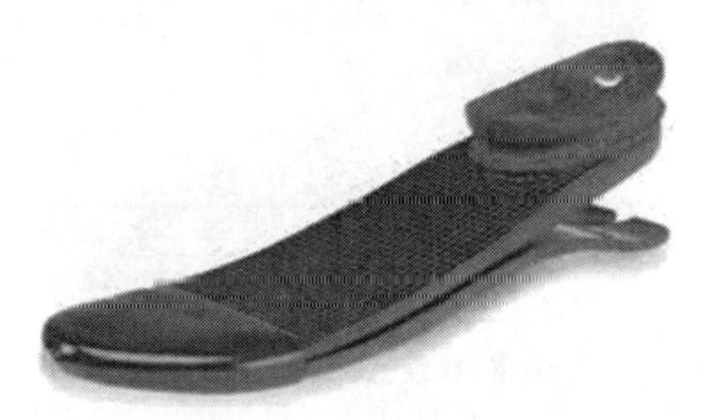

Figure 9.7 LP Symes foot, Freedom Innovations.

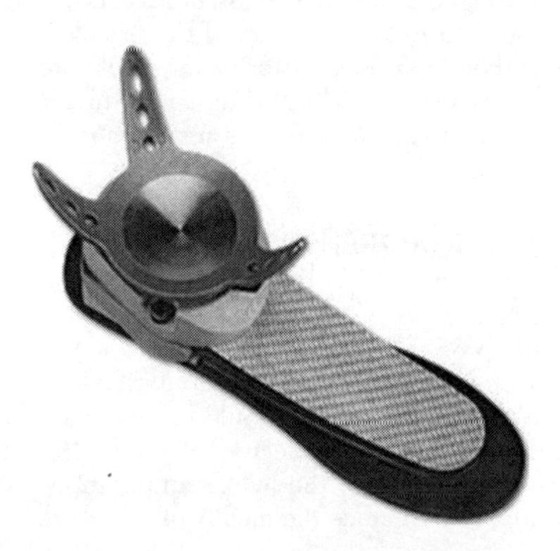

Figure 9.8 Otto Bock 1C90 ProSymes foot.

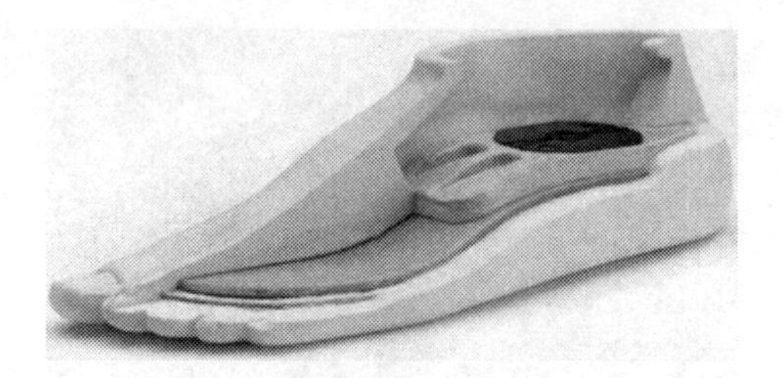

Figure 9.9 Willow Wood Carbon Copy Symes foot.

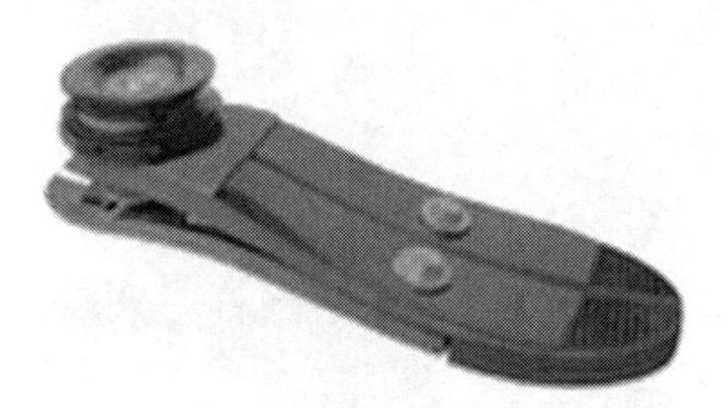

Figure 9.10 Ossur Flex-Symes foot.

more natural spring to the foot. The use of carbon fiber plates inside the footshell helps to reduce the bulk of the prosthesis at the ankle as well. The carbon fiber energy-storing low-profile feet are popular with younger active patients. The attachment of the foot to the socket is critical due to the stress placed on this area because of the long lever arm of the residual limb.

SYMES OR TRANSTIBIAL AMPUTATION?

This is a question no one can answer in a few words. One must consider all the pros and cons mentioned above for the individual patient to come to a conclusion on the amputation level. The benefits and downside of this amputation should be discussed fully with the patient and the family before a decision is made. Both the physical and prosthetic advantages of the Symes amputation are significant and can considerably enhance the quality of life for the amputee.

10

Transtibial Amputations

Patty Young

TRANSTIBIAL PROSTHETIC PRESCRIPTION

Prosthetic prescription can be challenging when taking all aspects of the patient into account: motivation level, prior level of function, current level of function, and personal goals for use of the prosthesis. Observing the patient's current level of activity in addition to reports by patient and family as to participation in therapies and hobbies reflecting motivation will give the practitioner an idea of the patient's ability to overcome obstacles, therefore providing insight into the likelihood of achieving goals. With these goals in mind, the practitioner can make a decision as to the shape of the socket, the material to be used for fabrication, and the appropriate prosthetic componentry.

Socket Design

There are two basic designs of transtibial (TT) sockets: patellar tendon bearing (PTB) and total surface bearing (TSB). It would be difficult to find a prosthetist who maintains the purity of either of these sockets, therefore creating a hybrid design, but it is through these theories that a design is chosen for a specific limb shape.

The PTB design is a pressure specific design allowing pressures in two specific areas: the patellar tendon bar and the posterior wall. The shape of this socket allows the residuum itself to be held off the bottom of the socket by the anterior–posterior pressures. The pressures capture the residuum at the patella bar level and maintain its' seated position on the patella bar using the forward pressure from the posterior wall. Patients are not always able to tolerate the sometimes aggressive pressures at the anterior and posterior aspects of the residuum and this may be the reason for the rejection of this design. It is important to note that the residual limb below the patellar tendon bar may not have contact with the socket interface in all areas and therefore, the wearer may feel a substantial amount of movement within the distal end of the socket.

The TSB socket is based on the true anatomical shape of the residuum with mild, if any, relief to the bony prominences. The pressures are more general and uniform throughout where no two areas are taking more pressure than anywhere else on the residuum. Volume management can be challenging as there tends to be overall volume reduction in a short period of time initially in this socket design, so the comfort of this socket type is dependent on the individual's ability to manage volume changes using varying sock ply. Hydrostatic socket design is a version of the TSB socket as it uses the theory of "full, uniform contact" but uses a casting method that applies uniform pressure around the entire residuum as the cast hardens and therefore controls the residuum by maintaining the same shape at any point in the gait cycle.

Socket Interfaces

The socket interface is the material between the socket and the residuum. An interface is used by a better part of the population of prosthetic wearers, but there are those who prefer not to utilize an interface as they tend to be seasoned users and skin breakdown is not of any concern to them. The most familiar type of interface is the pelite liner. The pelite liner is made from a foam-like material and is vacuum-formed to fit within the socket with the desired contours to prevent the residual limb from making contact with the hard socket. The lifespan of a pelite liner is between three and six months depending upon the wearer's activity level as the material can withstand only so much pressure before becoming thin and rendered ineffective.

Another form of interface has "flexible inner socket, hard outer socket" design. This implies that the prosthetist will fabricate the socket using a flexible thermoplastic material such as polypropylene, ipolen, or surlyn as the interface material. These materials are fabricated under an elevated vacuum system just as the pelite liner is but the integrity of this material does not "pack out" or become prematurely thin, and provides the prosthetist with the option of fenestrations in the hard outer socket. The flexible inner socket material also maintains its shape and contains the residuum true to form without becoming distended. As there are so many different materials out on the market that can be used for flexible inner sockets, the prosthetist determines the material based on the comfort required in the socket, the possibility for future fenestrations, and the flexibility of the material. A gel or silicone liner is also used as an interface between the socket and the residuum to provide comfort and protection to the residuum as well as control redundant tissue movement. This liner is made from a form of thermoplastic elastomer or silicone and is rolled onto the residuum while avoiding wrinkles. The liner should remain snug on the limb and the tacky inside of the liner prevents the liner from sliding off of the limb.

Suspension

Success in suspension will be determined by how the wearer interprets trust in the prosthesis. There are many ways to suspend the prosthesis but if there is much movement or displacement occurring within the socket during the gait cycle, the wearer will not feel the connection to the prosthesis required for good gait technique. There are many types of suspension to choose from and oftentimes, there is more than one appropriate option of suspension for an individual. The form of suspension should be based on many facets of the wearer. Does the individual have full strength and range of motion (ROM) of their hands to don/doff suspension sleeves or liners? Does the individual have intact vision? Does the wearer intend to participate in sports? Does the wearer have gadget tolerance? Is the individual's skin especially fragile? Are the habits of the wearer clean and hygienic?

Types of Suspension

The first type of suspension discussed is the supracondylar (SC) design which is used for both suspension and functional design on a PTB shaped socket. The SC design allows support to a short residuum or support for a limb with a poor ligamentous structure. Through high trimlines with very tactful modifications, the SC design also can provide anatomical suspension escaping the need for auxiliary suspension. The socket can be made with or without a suprapatellar (SP) bar which encompasses the patella itself and stops just proximal to it. The modifications in the fabrication process are specific and, when accurately done, will prevent genu recurvatum using the high trimline working as a kinesthetic reminder at mid-to-terminal stance.

This prosthetic socket choice was commonly used with a population of people, who performed frequent kneeling tasks, such as roofers and carpenters, but has since been replaced with more durable lay-up designs in fabrication to withstand the pressures. Suspension can also be attained through the use of the medial wedge, which requires fabrication flair. A medial wedge follows the contours just above the medial condyle and is removable during the donning/doffing process to allow the wearer to don with ease but feel "locked in" to the prosthesis.

The thigh corset with knee joint suspension is one of the oldest forms of suspension. The thigh corset, usually made of leather with eyelets and lacing, is fit to the individual and is worn at the lower two-thirds of the thigh. The knee joints are aligned to allow full knee range of motion but to prevent genu recurvatum and provide lateral and medial support for what may be a short residuum or a weak knee. As one can imagine, removing this prosthesis requires the wearer to remove their pants, which can be cumbersome and inconvenient, but there is a very faithful population of wearers who prefer to take the pressures of suspension and weight-bearing through the thigh corset rather than through the socket and avoid a TSB design.

The fork strap and belt suspension is another form of suspension, which is the longest used but also requires the wearer to don the prosthesis before putting pants on, making it difficult to remove without disrobing. The fork strap also utilizes a belt around the wearer's waist that runs along the anterior thigh and hooks onto a "y" strap on the medial and lateral trimlines of the socket. Since the socket is being suspended, in essence by the waist belt, the security in the suspension of the socket is often lacking for the wearer and therefore, this suspension cannot be used for high level activity or aggressive walkers.

Supracondylar cuffs are a common form of suspension with the generation of baby-boomers as this was a way of streamlining a fork strap without the need for the waist belt. The SC cuff is attached to the lateral and medial walls of the proximal aspects of the socket and connects to the limb just above the condyles using a circumferential strap. This form of suspension, when used for a long period of time, can create an indentation along the strap line and should be accompanied by education regarding what is "too tight" when tightening the strap as to not impede blood flow. The perception of proprioceptive feedback is better than in the thigh corset and fork strap with the waist belt, and the connection to the limb just over the condyles keeps the socket closer to the residuum.

A sleeve suspension secures the prosthesis to the individual's limb by use of a neoprene sleeve affixed to the prosthesis at the approximate midpoint of the socket and is rolled up the thigh and secured using circumferential strapping. This form of suspension should not be confused with a suction liner as it is not creating suction but rather, securing the prosthesis by sleeve alone. This type of suspension is often used as auxiliary suspension for activity specific limbs to ensure the least amount of displacement in the socket. The user must have good hand strength and ROM since the sleeve must be snug in fit in order to be effective.

In the 1980s came the development of the commonly known suspension using a pin-lock liner. This suspension has been used for those individuals with moderate visual and/or hearing impairments or those who perform heavy-duty tasks requiring the positive assurance that the pin-lock liner offers. These liners allow individuals the feedback and confidence to know that the suspension is secure and will not disengage. A liner, made of thermoplastic elastomer or silicone, has a pin secured to the center of the distal liner and is aligned with a lock fabricated into the socket. It is important to emphasize to the wearer the following: The liner *must be washed daily* to safeguard the liner from the growth of bacteria and therefore, the development of skin conditions causing breakdown in the skin on the residuum and potential for infection. The individual wearing the liner must have the hand strength to unroll and roll the liner into the correct position or should work with a physical therapist or occupational therapist to ensure that practice is involved in activities of daily living (ADL) training to enable the wearer to don/doff the liner without struggle. The challenge with wearing these liners comes at the beginning stages of wearing the prosthesis, as lining up of the pin as central on the distal residuum as possible will improve the ease with which the limb is donned and can often be frustrating for the new wearer since exact placement is so imperative. Care with donning must be practiced when wearing socks for volume management; should the socks fall within the lock mechanism, the lock will bind up and the prosthesis will not be released from the limb. A common report from wearers of a pin-lock suspension system is that the wearers feel the prosthesis pulling away from the limb in the swing phase of gait, and they often develop redundant tissue at the distal end of the residuum and/or breakdown at the distal anterior tibia.

The suction sleeve is another form of suspension requiring good hand strength and ROM as well as good hygiene. The suction sleeve is rolled over the liner or socks worn as an interface to the residuum and must be in contact with the skin of the thigh in order to create the closed suction suspension. A one-way valve is fabricated into the socket, usually at the most distal point, thus ensuring that any trapped air in the socket is expelled to provide an intimate fit. This suspension provides great proprioceptive feedback to the wearer but requires hygienic attention as the liner and sleeve should be cleaned and sanitized to ensure that bacterial growth does not occur. In addition to hygiene, the suspension sleeve is also susceptible to nicks and tears which will negatively change the efficacy of the suspension.

Suction suspension continues to be the gold standard for suspension but for those wearers who are tough on their outer suspension sleeve, a seal-in liner was created. This liner is made of silicone with a hypobaric sealing membrane (HSM) encircling the outside of the liner at the distal one-third. The wearer rolls the liner on as they would a regular gel liner and then sprays a mist of alcohol and water on the seal to decrease friction while sliding the residuum into the socket. A one-way expulsion valve is in the socket below the level of the HSM and a suction seal is created at the level of the HSM, thus generating suction suspension from the distal third of the residuum. The mist will dissipate locking the socket in place. This form of suspension is most suitable for those wearers who have been long time wearers and do not experience fluctuation in volume. This system of suspension does allow use of sock ply to address fit, but is not recommended for someone with volume changes greater than 5 ply sock thickness. When choosing the style of the seal-in liner, the prosthetist can choose a liner with either one HSM seal or five HSM seals depending upon the movement of the tissue within the socket and the need for supplemental suspension. For example, if a residuum has a strong remaining gastroc-soleus muscle belly, there will be moments in the gait cycle when the gastroc-soleus will contract therefore changing the general shape of the residuum and pulling the HSM away from the inner wall of the socket. In this example, the benefit of having a five-seal seal-in liner will ensure that suction is maintained despite the change in shape.

Finally, a form of suspension that is becoming more often used and seen in the younger population of wearers requiring a continued level of suspension throughout a variety of activities is the elevated vacuum system. There are several types of systems, but to refer to a suspension system as having "elevated vacuum," the system must maintain a certain amount of vacuum draw to prevent pistoning or movement within the socket. The basic lay-up of an elevated vacuum system requires a draw pump to draw air out of the socket pulling air from between the residuum and the inner socket to maintain the tissue against the walls of the socket at a desired level of vacuum within the confines of the socket, thus preventing movement in all directions. Most systems have been created so that the wearer and the prosthetist may select a desired amount of vacuum to be maintained triggering the device to turn on when such parameters have not been met. Elevated vacuum systems are user-friendly to a great extent; the wearer must understand the feel of the desired vacuum for appropriate suspension. Also, this suspension is not for those with inconsistent volume loss requiring frequent sock ply management.

Alignment

Alignment is the relationship between the socket, pylon, and the componentry, and the effect it has on the technique with which walking occurs. There are three types of alignment involved in all lower limb prosthetic setups: bench alignment or the standard starting alignment based on values recommended by the manufacturer, static alignment which takes into account the shift in alignment of the components with weight-bearing, and dynamic alignment where deviations are noted through the gait cycle. All three will be discussed with respect to a TT socket, a pylon and a prosthetic foot.

Bench alignment for the unilateral TT prosthesis starts from the sagittal plane. The socket is placed in 5 to 10 degrees of flexion to facilitate heel strike and to place the quadriceps complex on stretch. The foot position as seen in the sagittal plane is placed along the line of the anterior–posterior bisection of the socket directly along the lateral foot bolt in the SACH foot. From the coronal plane, the socket should be set in 2 to 5 degrees of adduction to protect the head of the fibula and to encourage a lateral shift at midstance along with the positioning of the foot medial to the bisection of the socket from a medial–lateral perspective. The inset or medial placement of the foot should be set with the reference point on the foot as the posterior bolt being placed medial to the bisection of the socket by one-half to one inch inset. Finally, the rotation of the foot should be accounted for in the coronal plane and is recommended at 3 to 5 degrees of external rotation to allow for smooth rollover from heel to toe. Bench alignment will vary in the bilateral TT setup in that recommendations for inset of the feet are now direct mid posterior foot in line with the bisection line of the socket to allow for a wider base of support and mild adduction in the sockets to prevent increased varus moment at midstance.

Static alignment in the unilateral TT is the time to look at the length of the prosthesis and the shift in the limb beneath the patient when the patient puts weight on the limb in the coronal plane. The base of support width should be 2 to 4 inches in width, the pylon should be vertical in orientation, and the hips should be level as noted when the clinician's hands are placed on the iliac crests. In the sagittal plane, the bisection of the socket should fall over the recommended point on the foot, be it the midpoint of the foot bolt or the distal one-third of the foot. The socket should remain in 5 to 10 degrees of flexion.

Dynamic alignment should be observed in a safe environment and is best observed with parallel bars and not with the use of assistive devices such as canes, walkers, or crutches. The practitioner should observe smooth rollover from heel to toe with good control of the knee, a consistent base of support width between two and four inches, toe clearance in swing phase, sound weight acceptance onto the prosthesis, level hips, and equal and consistent step length.

Prosthetic Feet

There are five basic types of prosthetic feet characterized by their ground reaction, movement (or lack thereof), and design. This section will review those starting from the least mobile, progressing to the most dynamic with indications for each foot.

The SACH foot is the first designed prosthetic foot and is designed with a **s**olid **a**nkle, **c**ushioned **h**eel, thus giving the foot its name. The keel is made of wood and in a fixed plantarflexed position of the foot with varying durometers of foam creating the cushioned heel. The durometer is chosen based on the wearer's weight as, the more the weight behind the heel strike, the more the compression creating a faster plantarflexion or "foot flat" moment. As one can probably imagine, most of the "movement" in this foot occurs at heel strike only, which makes up 5% of the gait cycle, and the remainder of movement must occur elsewhere in the wearer up the kinetic chain. SACH feet are appropriate for single cadence wearers whose greatest distances walked may be within the confines of the home where the terrain is flat and predictable and the required strain is minimized. This user is considered to be categorized as a K1 walker according to the Medicare Functional Classification Level (MFCL) or K Levels.

An elastic keel foot is the next version of prosthetic foot choice. This foot functions similarly to the SACH foot in that it is in a fixed position and achieves foot flat at heel strike-loading response into midstance based on the durometer of the heel. The keel of this foot, as it is elastic, enhances rollover in the gait cycle for those K1 walkers to prevent the knee, hip, and back from having to compensate for the lack of rollover in the SACH foot creating a smoother heel to toe motion. The elastic keel foot is lightweight and appropriate for light users but would not withstand an aggressive walker.

The single-axis foot allows immediate and definitive foot flat for the wearer upon heel strike to ensure stability into midstance. This type of foot is characterized by the foot bolt pivot point about which plantarflexion and dorsiflexion occur. Although a single-axis foot can be used by any prosthetic user, this foot is often chosen for those prosthetic wearers who have had an amputation at the transfemoral level and who require added stability to the prosthesis. By providing a patient with immediate foot flat, a knee extension moment is created with the plantarflexion moment of the foot thus making the knee a "safer" knee going into midstance. The single-axis foot adds material to the foot that can require maintenance or areas of potential breakdown, thus increasing the potential for a heavier and less maintenance-free foot than the SACH or elastic keel foot.

A multi-axial foot provides accommodation to the uneven terrain that the amputee negotiates in their daily activities. This foot, as with the single-axis foot, has more "parts" to the foot therefore making it a more customized option, but the need for maintenance and repair may increase based on the quality of the foot and the wearer's activity level. Through a series of bumpers, the multi-axial foot exhibits an ability to perform shock absorption for the wearer thus lessening the chance of breakdown of the residuum. The multi-axial foot used to be the gold standard for the K2 and K3 walkers and those who participate in outdoor activities, but in recent years, after a change in prosthetic design, many of the dynamic response feet accommodate for the frequent and unpredictable change in topography. This foot choice also tends to be a heavy alternative in feet therefore stressing the importance of effective suspension.

Finally, the dynamic response foot was created in the 1990s in order to "lighten the load" on the wearer by using carbon fiber material to provide an ultra-light, ultra-strong option for prosthetic feet. The design of the basic dynamic response foot is in the shape of a "J," which provides absorption of weight at heel strike, collection of energy from initial heel strike through midstance, and return of that energy at terminal stance from the congregated energy throughout the stance phase into the swing phase. Dynamic feet are for the K2 and K3 ambulators who will exhibit a change in cadence and require a foot to keep up with them. The "split toe" design of most dynamic response keels allow for medial/lateral terrain accommodation and a more natural heel to toe rollover since in normal human locomotion, the rollover begins at heel strike, progresses through the lateral border, and finishes medially pushing from the great toe.

11

Knee Disarticulation Prosthesis Criteria

John Fox

Knee disarticulation (KD) prosthesis affords a better distal end-bearing and suspension for the amputee. The two most common KD amputations are either with the condyles left untouched or beveled. Beveled condyles are more cosmetic in the finished prosthesis, but distal end-bearing areas, rotational control, and suspension are all sacrificed. When condyles remain, a KD amputation is superior to a transfemoral (TF) amputation except in cosmesis.

Trimlines should be more proximal than with a TF prosthesis to take advantage of distal end-bearing. The knee center of the fabricated prosthesis is lowered in the case of a KD, which leaves the floor-to-knee center shorter. This is evident, especially when the patient is sitting. The patient's foot will usually be 1 to 2 inches off the floor. The bulbous distal end, when enclosed in the liner and socket also makes the prosthesis less cosmetic.

Explaining these pros and cons to the amputee when evaluating for their prosthesis in a clinical setting decreases the anxiety of the patient and ensures greater acceptance of the prosthesis.

PRESCRIPTION CONSIDERATIONS AND OPTIONS

Years ago the socket for a KD was fabricated with molded leather and laced to accommodate circumferences and allow adjustments. This technique is rarely used today. The interface options are as follows.

Interface Options

Flexible Gel Liners With a One-Way Expulsion Valve (Suction)

Flexible gel liners add to the bulk of the distal end of the prosthesis and are less cosmetic than alternatives but offer an excellent form of suspension when used. A locking pin or a through-the-socket Velcro strap improves its function.

Multi-Durometer Materials

Multi-durometer interfaces made of materials such as pelite, plastazote, etc. also add bulk but allow ongoing inner socket adjustments to be made more easily and are more tolerant of skin surface issues (see Figure 11.1).

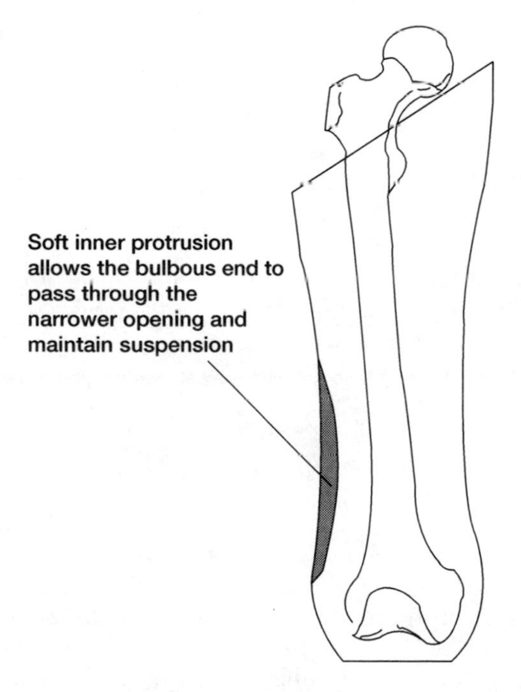

Figure 11.1 KD socket for use with a multi durometer liner.

Partial Suction

Partial suction uses a one-way expulsion valve and aids suspension.

Medial Door Opening

Medial door opening allows the bulbous distal end to pass through the narrower circumferences above the condyles and ensures a better suspension with its adjustability (see Figure 11.2).

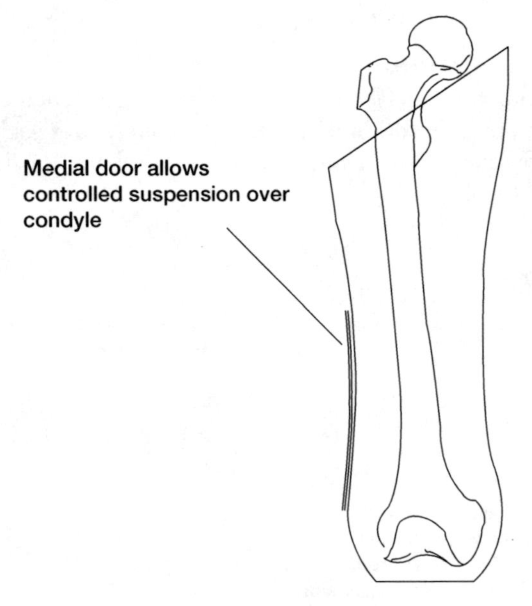

Figure 11.2 KD socket with medial opening and door.

These interfaces are some of the most commonly used. They can also be used in conjunction with each other.

KD Flexible Inner Liner With Rigid Frame

Knee disarticulation flexible inner liner with rigid frame permits custom design of the rigid frame to allow the bulbous distal end of the residual limb to pass through the narrower aspects of the socket. The inner liner is flexible and allows some expansion when donning.

Knee Selection

Polycentric

Polycentric knees (four-bar) offer the most cosmetic appearance. They allow the knee to more closely approximate the anatomical joint. The knee design is somewhat limited in range of motion (ROM) due to its design but is usually acceptable to the patient. These knees can incorporate a hydraulic or pneumatic unit and also provide good stability.

Microprocessor

Microprocessor knees (MPKs) are prosthetic knees with a processor/computer incorporated into it. These knees monitor and control the functions and capabilities of the prosthesis. Weight is a factor with these knees (6–7 lb). Maintenance requires a compliant patient.

Hydraulic/Pneumatic

Hydraulic/pneumatic knees control the flexion of the knee when the knee bends. This allows the patient to walk at various speeds as the cylinder increases/decreases the fluid or air contents.

Mechanical/Stance Phase

Mechanical/stance phase knees, often referred to as "stance control" knees, lock when weight is applied. These knees provide stability for the less active patients. Polycentric knees are the knee of choice for most KD prostheses. They provide better control during walking and the stance phase. These knees use multiple joints for stability adjustments. There has been a concentrated effort to bring all prosthetic knees closer to the anatomical knee center height. Historically this was not possible and KD prosthesis was constructed using outside metal joints along with the previously mentioned leather laced sockets. The shortened shank in most KD prostheses does not allow for accommodation of knees with longer build heights. Other knees are available for the KD prosthesis but the above knees are the ones most commonly used.

Prosthetic Feet for KD Prostheses

Non-Articulating (Flexible Keel)

Non-articulating feet are rigid and cannot bend, the heel compresses at weight-bearing, and the flexible forefoot allows rollover. The solid ankle cushion heel (SACH) foot is an example of a non-articulating foot.

Single Axis

Single-axis feet have joints that articulate up and down which aid in knee stability.

Multi-Axis

Multi-axis feet conform to more uneven surfaces and provide motion in multiple planes.

Dynamic Response

Dynamic response feet store and release energy. There are a multitude of these feet available, for various activities. They are often referred to as carbon feet or flex-feet.

Microprocessor Feet

Microprocessor feet monitor and control the functions and capabilities of the foot electronically as in the MPKs.

There are a multitude of prosthetic feet available commercially and different factors influence their choice. For example, the distance (build height) between the bottom of the knee component and the sole of the foot are usually shortened when fabricating a KD prosthesis. At times there is not enough build height to accommodate some of the prosthetic feet available.

Additional components, ie, rotators and shock absorbers, can be used as long as the build height allows. Prosthetic prescription for a KD prosthesis has to be a clinical team approach.

12

Transfemoral Prosthetic Prescription

Patty Young

Since the physicality of ambulating with a transfemoral prosthesis requires both endurance and strength, a person's prior level of function before amputation is a good determinant of the appropriateness for transfemoral prosthetic prescription before fabrication and success in future gait training on a prosthesis. The amputee care team should assess the patient's goals and the likelihood of achieving those goals before generating a prosthetic prescription for the future prosthetic wearer.

For example, in the transtibial population, making a limb for transfer assist is both safe and advantageous as it provides balance through the contact of the limb with the ground; this is not the case for transfemoral wearers. When an individual wears a transfemoral prosthesis, they are required to control both the knee joint and the foot/ankle joint thus making it a challenge for the wearer and the individual who is assisting with the transfer. The amputee care team should reinforce this to the patient to ensure full awareness and understanding that the knee will not lock unless the individual is in an erect, standing position and the standing position is not always required for safe transfers.

Safety is the emphasis in prosthetic prescription of the transfemoral prosthesis. The knee, in the most stable of prosthetics, will not lock unless the individual is in a full standing position and a hyperextension moment occurs to achieve knee extension lock. Since standing is required to don the prosthesis, steadying assist would be imperative for those patients who lack balance on a single limb. Another important factor to note: donning the transfemoral prosthesis requires a combination of sitting, supine, and standing in order to ensure the prosthesis is in correct alignment without clothing or undergarments inside the liner or socket and to prevent any anatomical discrepancies within the socket as well. With this in mind, donning a prosthesis requires standing balance and endurance of at least 5 minutes, and assist of a second individual if the new wearer has impairments in strength, endurance, balance, and cognition.

SOCKET DESIGN

The design of the transfemoral prosthetic socket is based on three factors: the anticipated activity level of the individual when the prosthesis is made, the tolerance to pressures on the ischial tuberosity and the ramus, and the amount of control the femur will require with respect to the strength of the muscles in the residuum. The three types of socket shapes are based on a combination of theory and practice and therefore rarely used in pure form.

The quadrilateral socket is a socket design from the 1950s created to enhance the whittled wooden socket. This socket uses a brim that is rectangular in shape with the medial and lateral walls being shorter than the anterior and posterior walls, and the ischial tuberosity and gluteal tissue seated on top of the posterior shelf. During the modification process, the anterior medial wall is flattened to apply gentle pressure in a broad manner along Scarpa's triangle to ensure the ischium remains on the flattened posterior ledge. This design lends itself to comfort for those who sit more than stand or ambulate.

The ischial containment (IC) socket came about in the 1980s in response to a more dynamic population of prosthetic wearers who were looking for control of the prosthesis through tissue containment and femur control. This socket design is recognized by the diamond shape of the socket when looking down on the socket and takes into account the full shape of the residuum through the casting process. The goal of this design is to control the femur's adduction for stability of the pelvis as well as control the tissue within the socket, thus controlling rotation of the socket. This design has a narrow medial–lateral measurement and a more open anterior–posterior measurement with well-crafted channels built into the socket for defined musculature, should it be present. The ischium in this socket is "contained" or enclosed within the socket on a more narrowly designed strut to encapsulate the ischium through the anterior medial and posterior lateral modifications made while fabricating the socket. It is important to note that the ischium should remain encapsulated by the strut in the swing phase and the stance phase to provide the wearer with the true feeling of control over the prosthesis.

A Marlo anatomical socket (MAS) is a ramal containment socket and is a form of IC socket design. This socket's design is a more challenging one to achieve and requires great skill in art and science to make this socket comfortable for the wearer. The design requires the medial wall of the socket to incorporate the ramus and the ischium with contours of the transition from the medial wall to the posterior wall without losing control of the ischium. This socket provides the wearer with a greater range of motion, but can be difficult to adjust to as the ramus is sensitive to pressures and is not often tolerated by everyone.

SOCKET INTERFACES

More common than in the transtibial socket, a flexible inner socket made from thermoplastics is often used in order to extend beyond the trimlines of the socket to prevent discomfort for the wearer. The material used to fabricate the flexible inner socket of the transfemoral socket is a flexible thermoplastic material. There are many versions of thermoplastic material, some with a smoother, slick finish often used for liners with lanyard straps and others with a tacky, gripping finish often used with true suction suspension or seal-in suspension. Pelite is not used in the transfemoral population since bony prominences are not an issue with a transfemoral prosthesis and therefore the flexible inner socket allows the wearer a more comfortable material to "sit on" or "sit in" to prevent direct contact with the acrylic resin, elevated vacuum formed carbon fiber–fiberglass outer socket. To make a transfemoral socket more comfortable for the wearer when sitting, fenestrations are created in the hard outer socket allowing the posterior tissue, ie, the hamstrings, to relax out of the hard outer socket and be contained within the flexible inner socket.

METHODS OF SOCKET SUSPENSION

There are many ways to suspend a prosthesis as seen in the transtibial prosthetic prescription chapter, but suspension in the transfemoral prosthesis requires more containment of tissue and less assist in suspension from bony prominences. The suspension of a transfemoral prosthesis is as imperative as that of the transtibial prosthesis, but the weight of the knee component, as well as the shorter lever arm of the residuum will truly affect the success with the prosthesis when the time for gait training comes.

The Silesian belt is secured to the socket at the lateral wall and then wraps around the individual's waist above the contralateral iliac crest fastening itself to the anterior socket that is situated at an angle toward the contralateral iliac crest. The belt is effective in controlling rotation within the socket and will not be affected by the addition of socks. The total elastic suspension (TES) belt is usually made of neoprene that is secured to the socket through its narrow design to fit snuggly around the socket, and then extends up the lateral aspect of the hip on the prosthetic side and fastening around the pelvis/hips bilaterally. Both of these belts allow the individual to feel a more secure connection with the prosthesis, but the connection of the prosthesis with the body is at the hips instead of at the residuum, which can throw the prosthetic wearer off when it comes to proprioception. The TES belt also tends to increase the likelihood of sweating as the material does not breathe and fits snugly against the body and some feel the need to remove the belt when using the restroom. This type of suspension is often used as supplemental suspension for high activity limbs.

A hip joint and pelvic band is a form of suspension similar to the Silesian belt with the difference being in the placement of the hip joint. The joint is attached to the socket at the most proximal aspect of the lateral wall of the socket and has an attached piece, usually made of plastic, which is contoured to the wearer's ipsilateral pelvis just below the iliac crest. The pelvic band is made of leather and extends from the contoured piece wrapping around the contralateral hip and fastening anteriorly. The hip joint and pelvic band have been used for extremely short residuums that do not have the lateral/abductor strength in order to create stability in midstance.

As seen in transtibial prosthetics, liners are used as forms of suspension through either a lanyard Velcro strap or a pin-lock design. These liners are similar to those used in transtibial prosthetics except for a difference in shape to better fit the transfemoral residual limb. The use of a liner can be a very concrete way of donning/doffing a prosthesis providing the wearer with comfort in the security of the suspension. The undesirable situation with this suspension is the increased likelihood of uncontrolled rotation where no number of socks can control for the rotation, should the volume of the residuum decrease while ambulating.

A seal-in liner, also discussed in transtibial suspension, is frequently seen in the mature transfemoral residual limb. Using seal-in suspension, the wearer has control over pistoning movement within the socket as well as rotational movement within the socket, thus preventing issues with breakdown. Sock ply management must be carefully attended to in order to perfect the fit of the socket to enhance proprioception and control of the prosthesis. A one-way valve is used for expelling pocketed air to secure the suction from the hyperbaric membrane at the distal third of the liner and limb.

True suction is the gold standard of transfemoral prosthetic suspension, although not always the best choice for every patient. This suspension is for the mature limb, where weight fluctuation is not a common occurrence and sufficient adipose tissue and muscle are available. True suction provides the most intimate level of fit and the best proprioceptive feedback than in any other suspension technique. It requires the wearer's bare skin to maintain contact with the flexible inner socket of the prosthesis in close quarters without areas of pocketed air through the use of a one-way valve to allow the release of excess air to maintain suspension. As one can imagine, donning would be difficult, given the friction between bare skin and a tacky inner socket, and there are many ways in which a wearer can don the prosthesis to achieve suction. One way to don the prosthesis for true suction is to use a lubricating agent, such as liquid powder, lotion, or alcohol–water combination (50/50); the lubricant is applied to the residuum to allow the limb to slide frictionless into the socket, and after several minutes and through expulsion of the excess air out of the one-way valve, the socket will create a suction lock on the residuum. The benefits of using a lubricant are the ease of use and the accessibility to the alcohol–water or lotion; these lubricants can clog up the one-way valve, though, requiring a new valve as suction cannot be maintained. Using materials such as ace wrap or a pull bag designed with a double-thickness material similar to parachutes allows the wearer to put their entire limb into the socket first, and then to remove the ace wrap or the pull bag, via the valve hole while establishing suction.

SOCKET ALIGNMENT

Alignment of the transfemoral socket requires proper alignment of the knee and the foot with respect to the pelvis and the femur to facilitate efficient, safe gait technique. In bench alignment, the frontal view is where the adduction, lateral/medial orientation of the foot, and the rotation orientation of the knee and foot occur. Adduction is determined by what is already present in the femur (known as Long's Line) plus adding 2° to 5° of adduction depending upon the length of the femur and the strength of the controlling muscles of the femur. The foot should be outset by 1 inch from the ischium-to-floor plumb line to allow for lateral weight shift onto the limb at midstance and 5° of external rotation should be accounted for at the knee joint for ease of swing phase. Bench alignment in the sagittal view should be driven by the trochanter-knee-ankle (TKA) line which follows a plumb line to align the trochanter over the center of the knee bolt and both the trochanter and the knee bolt over the foot at a specified area set by the manufacturer for proper alignment. Static alignment is assessed when the patient is wearing the limb and before ambulating to ensure all alignment specifications are correct when in a weight-bearing position. It is during static alignment that changes are made using an offset plate for flexion accommodations in the hip and the pyramid is used for angular changes to encourage weight shifting in both the coronal and sagittal planes. Dynamic alignment is observed when walking in a safe environment, often parallel bars, during which gait deviations are identified and changes made for more efficient gait technique.

PROSTHETIC KNEES

When choosing a prosthetic knee, strength and balance should drive the choice of knee componentry. Safety is imperative and the patient's knee choice needs to reflect the strength and cognition in controlling the mechanics of the knee. Knees are identified by their level of stability and safety. Below, knee types are discussed from the greatest level of stability to lesser inherent stability.

Locking Knee

The locking knee is the most stable of all knees as the locking mechanism prevents the knee from flexing at any time during the gait cycle. The individual needs to be trained in the use of the lock in order to release it when going from a standing to a sitting position and engage it when standing up from a seated position. The benefit of this type of knee is a secure, locked, stable knee, but the disadvantages are that the straight leg position greatly affects the gait technique and the efficiency in gait, as circumduction and hip hiking are required on the prosthetic side.

Four-Bar Polycentric Knee

The four-bar polycentric knee is the next knee described as "inherently stable." The stability of this knee is in its design in that the alignment within the knee creates stability and the alignment of the knee within the total alignment of the prosthesis is stable, therefore providing security and stability while providing ease of swing into flexion from an extended position. The advantage of this knee is that it will bend with weight-bearing through the forefoot or toe and will lock with the swing phase for security when placing weight through the heel. Given the design of the knee, the prosthesis in flexion during the initial and the mid-swing phase will shorten the shank making it an ideal knee for those with a knee disarticulation when attempting to keep the knee center close to the same height as the sound limb. The disadvantage is the potential for maintenance on the knee; given the number of hinges and articulations and the potential for the wearer to create a gait cycle with a "goose-stepping" tendency: kicking the knee out hard and fast and slamming the heel of the foot down for security going in to stance phase.

Stance Control Knee

The stance control knee is the next stable knee in the line-up of prosthetic knee choices. This type of knee, as implied in the name, allows for control of the stability of the knee when in a weight-bearing position through a clutch-lock design, but it should be emphasized that this knee requires a certain amount of weight to secure the clutch-lock. The new amputee will not yet have developed prosthetic trust and therefore often does not shift weight onto the prosthesis in order to activate the clutch-lock knee during the stance phase, and will experience unwanted knee flexion if not careful. The need to remove all weight from the prosthesis at terminal stance presents a challenge when the wearer is attempting to flex the knee in order to allow the knee to bend. This is obvious when sitting as the wearer must shift all weight off of the prosthesis and use the sound limb only to lower the amputee onto the seat of the chair. As the disadvantage is the need for weight-bearing in order to create trust, this too, can be the advantage as practitioners struggle in training patients to trust in the prosthetic side and by encouraging the only way to create the "brake" effect of the knee to prevent flexion is to shift full weight onto the limb for stability. Another advantage is the ease of swing in this prosthetic knee to initiate flexion preventing accessory motion at the hip and torso.

Constant Friction, Single-Axis Knee

The constant friction, single-axis knee is a knee moving away from stability and closer to improved voluntary swing features. The constant friction feature of the knee reveals the fixed cadence feature of the knee most noted in the swing phase of the gait cycle. The single-axis design is that of a hinge, similar to the knee joint as it allows rotation of the joint around one and only one junction. The advantages of the constant friction, single-axis knee are the durability and reliability of the knee. The disadvantage of this knee is the fixed cadence. The wearer is required to have the strength to control the knee at any point in the gait cycle, should the knee be triggered by the ground or by weight shift in the wrong direction; this is why it is imperative that the alignment of this knee is accurate and the knee is set up in safe alignment.

Fluid-Controlled Knees

Fluid-controlled knees are the final category of knees on the market in prosthetic choice. These knees have a cylinder with a piston and the fluid; either air (pneumatic) or a liquid (hydraulic) passes through the piston creating a varied cadence in swing allowing the wearer to increase or decrease their speed without lag time of the knee. The disadvantages of these knees are in the weight and the expense and therefore should be used for those who will be capable of ambulating with a varied cadence. Maintenance should also be considered when prescribing the fluid-controlled knees to a patient as the piston needs to be serviced annually and care should be taken to store the knee in an upright position whenever the prosthesis is not in use.

Microprocessor Knees

Following the ideas and concepts of the fluid-controlled knees, microprocessor knees came into use in the mid-1990s in an effort to enhance the intelligence and safety of the fluid-controlled knee. Each company manufacturing a microprocessor knee uses the basic hydraulic concept controlled by sensors receiving information based on the position of the knee and the ground reaction forces in order to determine the safest position of the knee. These knees are expensive and require the user to have gadget tolerance in order to successfully use the knee. The safety features of these knees make them desirable for any user in the K3 level. There are attempts in some microprocessor knees to appeal to the K2 walker as safety is imperative for all ambulators with a prosthesis, but not all insurance companies are willing to supply funding for microprocessor knees in this population.

PROSTHETIC FEET

Prosthetic feet do not differ from those selected in the transtibial prescription, so please refer to the transtibial prescription chapter. Do note though, the single-axis foot is commonly prescribed for the initial training prosthesis as it allows immediate foot flat without excessive multi-axial movement giving the walker a sense of security when in contact with the ground. Remember, when prescribing a multi-axial or dynamic response foot, the wearer must have good pelvic control and control of the socket in order to feel secure since medial lateral movement greatly effects the perception of balance.

STUBBIES

Stubbies are used when training an individual with bilateral transfemoral amputations and the use of stubbies is controversial amongst prosthetists and therapists alike. The stubby set-up consists of sockets, short pylons and uniquely designed "stubby feet." The sockets are traditionally designed with an ischial containment shape for comfort as the quad socket design would be too cumbersome medially. The length of the pylon is set to achieve the height of the average seat of a chair within the rehab environment. The stubby feet are found in two shapes: triangular, where the base of the triangle is turned posteriorly and the pylon is mounted on the tip, and in the shape of a bean, where the pylon is mounted one-third of the length of the bean and the longer aspect of the bean is turned posteriorly. The reason the stubby feet are created with more surface area facing posteriorly is to allow some push back when the new amputee is learning to find their balance as leaning posteriorly would result in falling backwards versus falling forward where one can extend their arms for support.

The theory behind the use of stubbies is based on the idea of creating and establishing a sense of balance on limbs without any articulating joints, such as feet or knees, allowing the new amputee to adjust to walking on "stilts." Over time and with an improvement in balance and strength, the wearer is progressed by lengthening the pylons first moving the center of mass away from the floor. The next step involves replacing the stubby feet with traditional prosthetic feet. Finally, the knees are introduced in the set up according to the individual's balance and strength, and oftentimes, one at a time.

Challenges with the rehabilitation process lie in the location in which the training occurs. The setting is imperative as the environment requires parallel bars and other supportive equipment such as harnessing for ambulation and transfer training to afford the amputee the sense of security and safety. If the individual were to return home with stubbies before training, the height of beds, chairs and other surfaces at home may be too high for the individual to transfer onto. As the patient progresses and the stubbies are lengthened, modifications and compensation may be made to the home to make the environment more accessible with the stubbies. All in all, the rehab process can be timely but effective for this population, given the motivation of the wearer.

13

Hip Disarticulation, Hemipelvectomy Amputation, and Prostheses

Terry L. Kalter

THE SURGERY

The technique of hip disarticulation is an amputation through the hip joint capsule, removing the entire lower extremity, with closure of the remaining musculature over the exposed acetabulum. Boyd attempted to minimize blood loss by transecting muscles at either their origin or insertion, these areas being relatively avascular. A higher level of amputation in this region is the hemipelvectomy which consists of removal of the entire lower extremity as well as all or a major portion of the ilium.

CAUSES

The major causes of hip disarticulation amputation are osteosarcoma, diaphyseal tumors and trauma. In the past, for fear of recurrence, hip disarticulation was the chosen treatment of distal femoral osteosarcomas. This was prior to the induction of chemotherapy and radiation therapies in the 1970s. Today 90% of these are treated without amputation at all. Amputations performed for vascular disease are often on a semi-emergency basis. The typical patient is in sepsis from multiple failed above-knee procedures or clotted femoral–popliteal grafts. Hemipelvectomy amputations are performed for the treatment of malignant tumors about the hip and pelvis.

POST-AMPUTATION

Patients are routinely transferred to a rehabilitation hospital immediately after surgery for a 2-week period of intensive therapy. Patients are instructed in the use of crutches and a walker, and are taught how to wrap their stump. This, in conjunction with a support group for amputees and sarcoma patients, has been found to be beneficial. Early and intensive psychological and physical rehabilitation results in most patients being completely independent and ambulatory at the end of one year.

Prosthetic fitting is typically limited to those patients that are motivated and physically fit. Good balance is necessary to don and ambulate with a prosthesis. The energy requirements to use this high level prosthesis can be as much as 200% of normal ambulation.

The lack of muscle power at the hip, knee, and ankle/foot results in a fixed, slow cadence. Many amputees at these higher levels find it easier to use crutches without a prosthesis. The prosthesis may be heavy, and difficult to learn to use.

THE PROSTHESIS

The prosthetic component selection and alignment for hip disarticulation and hemipelvectomy are quite similar. Stability is built into the prosthesis by having the weight line fall anterior to the knee center in the sagittal plane.

The traditional device prior to 1954 consisted of a molded leather socket with a laterally placed locking hip joint called a tilt-table prosthesis. The lateral placement tried to approximate the anatomical location of the hip joint.

The "Canadian" design with an anterior placed hip joint was introduced in 1954. This design used an unlocked hip, knee, and ankle joint that relied on biomechanics to achieve stance-phase stability while permitting flexion at the hip and knee during the swing phase. This design results in a significantly shortened prosthesis to prevent the amputee from vaulting for toe clearance.

The Hip Joint

For many years, modular hip joints like those below were the only ones commercially available. This is most likely due to the small number of this higher level of amputations performed.

7E4 – Otto Bock Modular Single-Axis Hip Joint, With Extension Assist

This hip joint has a lateral mounted latex band as a hip joint extension assist (see Figure 13.1). This limits the range of motion during the swing phase of gait. Transverse rotation and adjustable extension stop are the only adjustments available.

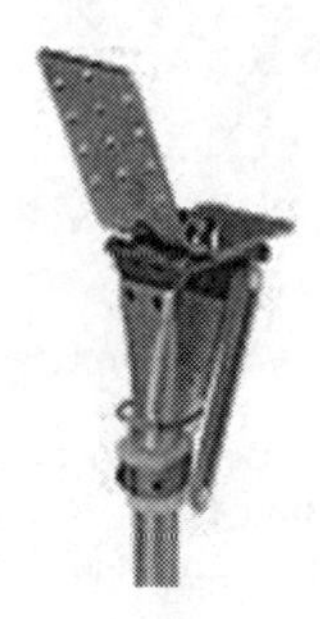

Figure 13.1 7E4 – Otto Bock modular single-axis hip joint, with extension assist.

7E5 – Otto Bock Modular Single-Axis Hip Joint, With Lock

This hip joint is locked in full extension and must be manually unlocked for sitting (see Figure 13.2). Transverse rotation is the only adjustment available.

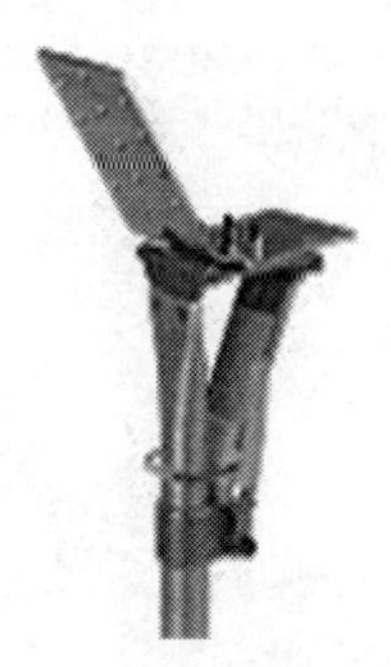

Figure 13.2 7E5 – Otto Bock modular single-axis hip joint, with lock.

7E7 – Otto Bock Adjustable Abduction/Adduction, Flexion/Extension, Extension Assist

This hip joint almost exclusively replaced the two modular hip joints above due to its increased adjustability (see Figure 13.3). It offers abduction/adduction, flexion/extension adjustments as well as transverse rotation. There is also an adjustable internal extension assist.

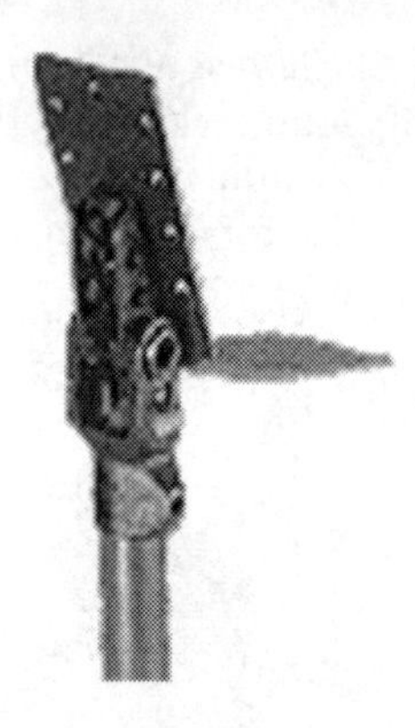

Figure 13.3 7E7 – Otto Bock adjustable abduction/adduction, flexion/extension, extension assist.

Otto Bock Helix Hip Joint

A newer hip joint option is the Helix hip joint by Otto Bock (see Figure 13.4).

It uses springs that store energy during the stance phase and releases this energy during swing to compensate for missing hip flexor muscles. It also uses hydraulics to dampen hip extension at heel strike. The Helix hip joint produces a three-dimensional hip movement to compensate for pelvic rotation and promotes a symmetrical and natural gait pattern. There is an improved sitting posture, a reduced pelvic obliquity, and a large flexion angle, which

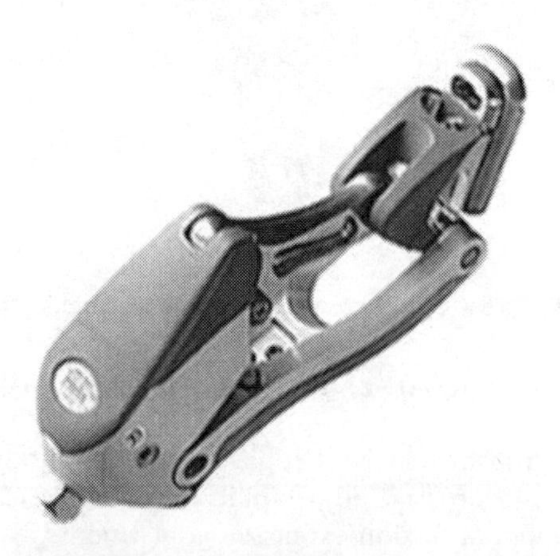

Figure 13.4 Otto Bock Helix hip joint.

make it easier to accomplish activities of daily living such as putting on shoes or getting into a car. It only has a maximum patient weight of 220 lbs and must be used with Otto Bock knees and feet for warranty purposes.

Another hip joint option is the Otto Bock four-bar knee disarticulation joint mounted in reverse. As with any polycentric knee, there is increased ground clearance during the swing phase due to the inherent "shortening" of the unit in flexion, enhanced stability at heel strike, and good appearance while sitting.

Carbon composite strut systems are available that offer more dynamic motion.

The Knee Joint

The single-axis (constant-friction) knee remains the most widely utilized due to its lightweight, low cost, and excellent durability. A low friction setting is used to ensure full knee flexion at terminal swing. The weight activated brake stance control (safety) knee is another commonly used knee for these higher amputation levels. This is the knee of choice for many prosthetists and therapists due to the independent adjustable friction; it is adjustable up to 15° at which the knee will not buckle when weight is applied. This makes ambulation safer in misstep situations. The problem with this knee is that weight has to be eliminated for the knee to become free in the swing phase. Weight also has to be transferred to the sound side and the prosthesis unweighted to sit. These knees cannot be used bilaterally because both knees cannot be unweighted simultaneously for sitting.

The polycentric or four-bar knee unit is another knee option for this higher level of amputation. Due to the inherent stance stability design, it shortens upon flexion for toe clearance during swing. The use of a manual locking knee is contraindicated due to the need for one hand to unlock the knee for sitting, which has proven to be too unstable. Fluid control knees (hydraulic or pneumatic) are not used because these patients ambulate at a fixed cadence.

The Foot

Solid ankle cushion heel (SACH) feet can be used for these amputation levels as well. A soft heel should be used to increase knee stability at heel strike. A single-axis foot with a soft plantarflexion bumper can also be used. Multi-axial feet offer the benefits of inversion/eversion and transverse rotation. This enables the patient to traverse uneven ground better and reduces shear forces on the residuum.

Although single-axis and multi-axial feet may be used to increase stability, they add substantial weight, cost, and maintenance.

Feet with a flexible keel, offer a softer, more flexible forefoot that results in a smoother rollover for the patient. Examples of these feet are the solid ankle flexible endoskeleton (SAFE), the Sten, and the dynamic foot.

Dynamic response feet are commonly chosen because they provide active push-off which is extremely beneficial during a more rapid gait.

Torque absorbers can be added just below the knee to reduce the stress on the residuum and may somewhat compensate for normal rotation during ambulation.

Transverse-rotation units placed proximal to the knee joint allow the patient to rotate the knee/shank/foot complex to maneuver in tight areas like getting into or out of a car, or sitting cross-legged.

Whatever foot is chosen, we must not forget the relationship it has with the knee joint. The more the motion in the foot, the more the stability required in the knee mechanism.

The Socket

A good fitting socket is critical to enable the patient to control the prosthesis. It must incorporate comfortable axial support and suspension. It must provide anterior–posterior stability to control rotation and allow active lumbar lordosis using the muscles of the lower back and abdomen during ambulation. All soft tissue should be used for axial loading and/or stability. Relief needs to be provided for bony prominences notably the pubis, iliac crests, and anterior superior iliac spines. In the hip disarticulation prosthesis, the ischial tuberosity should be used for weight-bearing. It is important to view x-rays to know what part of the skeletal anatomy is remaining. It is sometimes difficult to know what lies underneath the soft tissue relying on palpation alone. Suspension during the swing phase is achieved by medial–lateral pressure above the iliac crests.

The most commonly used socket material is a rigid thermosetting resin which may be polyester, acrylic, or epoxy. Comfort can be increased using a flexible thermoforming inner socket and an external rigid frame. There are also custom liners made out of silicone or polyurethane gel that will further increase comfort. The more comfortable the patient is in the socket, the more apt they are to be a functional prosthetic user.

CONCLUSION

The success of fitting a hip disarticulation or hemipelvectomy prosthesis is dependent upon a socket that is comfortable, flexible, and correctly aligned. Early fitting also increases the acceptance of a prosthesis for these higher levels of amputation. We as health care providers must evaluate each case independently as they are all individuals with unique desires and capabilities.

14

Prosthetic Considerations for Patients With Partial Hand Amputation

Allison Hickman

Amputation distal to the wrist joint is one of the most common amputations. Amputation of the fingers represents the largest portion of these (74%) and of the thumb the second most common at 16% [1]. Unfortunately, partial hand amputations are one of the most difficult to fit with a prosthesis. This is due to many factors including suspension challenges, loss of proprioception, aesthetics, and discomfort at the prosthesis–body interface. In the past, when only cosmetic or bulky mechanical units were readily available, the vast majority of partial hand amputees elected to go without a prosthesis [2]. With newer technologies becoming more common and accessible, however, more partial hand amputees have access to practical prosthetic devices. Advances in materials, suspension, mechanics, and prosthesis–body interface have also introduced more options for the partial hand amputee to facilitate return to vocational and recreational activities integral to the physical and psychosocial well-being of the amputee.

The physiologic complexity of the upper extremity, and the hand specifically, creates a significant challenge for prosthetic management for both the patient and the prosthetist. Additionally, aside from the etiology of amputation, the personal experiences and perceptions of the amputee will play a significant role in prosthetic evaluation, implementation, and utilization. Patient factors such as personality, stage of life, prior functional ability, cognitive ability, and social support networks should greatly influence prosthetic selection. Hand dominance and vocational and recreational goals should also be considered in the decision process. As such, a team approach involving the patient, the patients' therapist, prosthetist, and medical providers (to address pain, skin, or surgical issues) is ideal when evaluating a patient for a partial hand prosthesis.

Approximately 75% of acquired amputation of the upper extremity is due to trauma [3]; 90% of finger loss and 82% of thumb loss are attributable to trauma [1]. Levels of amputation include finger (transphalangeal) occurring at the distal interphalangeal joint, proximal interphalangeal joint, or metacarpaphalangeal levels. Transmetacarpal amputation and wrist amputation are less commonly seen because they typically have decreased functional outcomes and the decision to take the amputation to the more functional transradial level is a common occurrence. Though the nature of the trauma will in part dictate the level of amputation, careful surgical consideration of the amputation level is also necessary to preserve maximum function. This can be especially true due to current advances in surgical limb salvage techniques where residual tissues, including that in patients with burns and grafts, may be especially vulnerable to pressure and traction from a prosthesis, and/or be especially sensitive or alternatively insensate. For some patients, surgical reconstruction of the hand may be more appropriate in order to preserve sensation and maximize function without a prosthetic device. It is typically accepted that there is little advantage to preservation of a partial hand without a thumb or metacarpals in that prosthetic fitting and use would be exceptionally difficult.

When assisting a patient with the selection of a prosthesis for partial hand amputation, three related goals should be considered and addressed. The primary goal should be prosthetic fit to the patient's residual limb. As with all prosthetic devices, advanced functional characteristics of the device itself are useless if the patient cannot comfortably wear the prosthesis. Appropriate fit must consider the shape and contour of the residual limb, skin integrity, degree of retained sensation, and degree of residual range of motion. A prosthesis will exert non-anatomical pressures and shear upon the residual limb, an aspect that can be especially important to consider in patients with altered sensation. Bimanual stability is the second goal, with restoration of functional prehension the third. The patient should be able to grossly manipulate an object using the prosthesis and the opposite functional hand (or the opposite prosthesis in cases of bilateral amputation). The ability for bimanual manipulation depends significantly on the patient's ability to control a prehensile grip with the prosthesis.

As stated earlier, the decision of whether to use a prosthesis and what type of device, will ultimately depend on the patient's needs and the recommendations of an amputee rehabilitation team. As with all prosthetic devices, needs will also change with time (natural reshaping of the residuum as it heals/becomes accustomed to prosthetic use), with the patient's desired activity level (vocational and recreational demands) and ability level (needs may dictate change in device weight, technological complexity, device power, etc.). Selection and interval evaluation of the amputee and their chosen device(s) are extremely important for patient safety, residual limb health, sound limb health, and to maximize function.

OVERVIEW OF PROSTHETIC OPTIONS FOR THE PARTIAL HAND AMPUTEE

Due to the variation in types of partial hand amputation, the amputee has several options when it comes to prosthetic selection. These include passive non-functional prostheses, passive functional prostheses, and active functional prostheses (including cable driven and powered devices). It should be noted, however, that even a passive non-functional prosthesis usually does perform more of a role than simply cosmesis in that it can be used to push or balance an object against the body or the opposite limb. Alternatively, and for a multitude of reasons, the amputee may choose to not use a prosthesis at all. Many studies have found that partial hand amputees will only wear their prosthesis when at work or in public to decrease attention drawn to the amputated limb.

A passive non-functional prosthesis is typically fashioned out of medium density foam or lightweight wood and covered with a polyvinyl chloride (PVC) or silicone cover to give variable life-like appearances of the limb. As stated above, this category is a bit of a misnomer in that an amputee missing a digit but retaining the metacarpophalangeal joint can use a passive finger prosthesis to be quite functional with the aid of the remaining intact digits of the hand. Due to the simplicity of these prostheses, and depending on the materials used, cost can be significantly controlled.

For amputees who are only missing a thumb and maintain a functioning first metacarpophalangeal joint, a passive opposition post, with or without a cosmetic cover, is typically recommended. This configuration allows for a highly functional "three-jaw chuck" grip pattern. In amputees who retain an intact thumb, even if the remainder of the metacarpals is shortened, a passive prosthetic device is often fitted to act as a post against which the unaffected thumb can oppose. In general, it is only in those patients in whom the thumb and all four fingers are lost at or proximal to the metacarpophalangeal joint is an active functional hand prosthesis recommended.

A passive functional prosthesis provides no active movement but can be configured with various internal components that can be positioned using the sound hand to provide many grasp patterns [4]. The hand may be rigid, have positionable fingers, or spring loaded grasp mechanism. These prostheses can allow the amputee to perform many tasks such as stabilizing or pushing against an object. In fact, past studies have shown that partial hand amputees who use a passive hand prosthesis use their prosthesis more than those fitted with active functional units [5]. The passive prosthesis generally includes a suction type total contact socket with the goal of providing a secure fit. The functional "joints" are held in place by manual locks or by friction once they have been moved into the desired position.

Active functional prostheses for the partial hand amputee will ideally allow for the maximum number of functional grip patterns including pincer (three-jaw chuck), tip (precision), spherical, lateral ('key grip'), and cylindrical (power grasp). The three-jaw chuck is the most commonly used and most versatile of the gripping patterns, and the majority of terminal devices take advantage of this grip pattern as their primary function. This gripping pattern can be performed with a two-prong hook, a greifer, or with finger-like extensions. When the latter is used (like the VASI and RSL Steeper MultiControl™ Plus hands by Liberating Technologies and the System Cable and Electric Hands by Otto Bock) the lateral or "key grip" function can be incorporated into a hand that performs the three-jaw chuck pattern by allowing the prosthetic thumb to go from an adducted (pincer) position to an abducted (lateral grip) position. In all but a few advanced powered devices, this position change is performed with the aid of the sound limb and the joint is held in place by manual lock or friction.

For amputees with partial hand amputation, there are two body-powered options available to activate the terminal device: cable driven and wrist or finger driven devices. Inherent disadvantages of cable driven devices include harness discomfort and the fact that force actuation, and therefore pincer or grip pressure, is dependent on the patient's ability to operate the cable system. Also, using a cable system requires atypical joint movements (usually at the shoulder) to activate the terminal device. This not only calls attention to the amputee when the terminal device is being activated but can also lead to

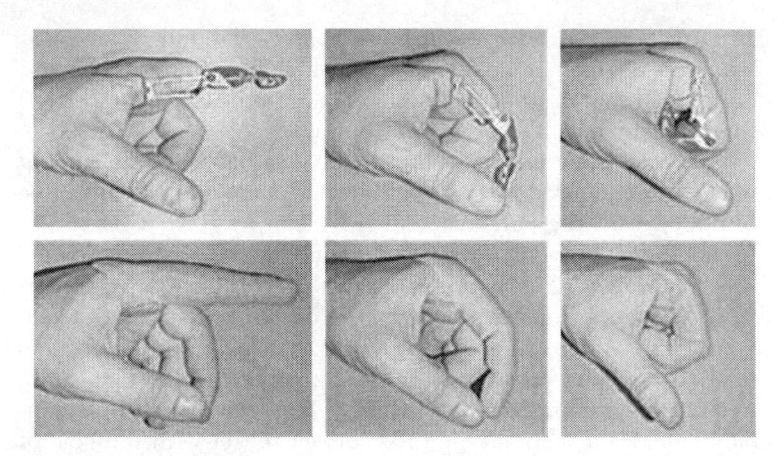

Figure 14.1 X-finger.
***Source*: From Dedrick Medical, Naples, FL. Used with permission.**

joint and muscle overuse injuries. The X-finger and the X-thumb by Dedrick Medical (Figure 14.1) are examples of finger driven devices and will be discussed later. Wrist driven units require the patient to be able to flex and extend the wrist to activate the device effectively creating a synthetic tenodesis pincer grasp. The force of the grasp will depend on not only the strength of the patient but also the functional range of motion of the joint used to generate the force.

Externally powered prostheses, until recently, were not practical for partial hand applications due to the bulk of components to perform complex and synergistic finger movements. Newer technology using smaller, more powerful, and more energy efficient motors and actuators now make it possible to incorporate external power into compact and more life-like terminal devices including individual fingers, all fingers and the thumb. Externally powered devices are still powered by the patient; however, an external power source (battery) is used to transform and/or amplify the given signal (input) to operate the terminal device. Due to the availability of residual forearm musculature in most partial hand amputees, a proportional myoelectric signal transducer is the most common input source used for externally powered partial hand prostheses. The ideal source of control for an externally powered prosthetic device will depend on the functionality of the amputees' remaining anatomy. Ideally, the control device will have two inputs: one for opening the finger(s) and one for closing them. For partial hand amputees the input sources are typically over muscles that would normally activate the desired motion in an intact hand. Though these devices do provide the amputee with a more realistic representation of the human hand and its function, significant limitations for their use continue to exist. Due to their intricate nature, fully myoelectric terminal devices are not well-suited for heavy lifting or for wet or dirty environments. They require batteries that must be recharged daily to every few days, and programming, general maintenance, and repair require special, typically proprietary, training, and expertise. Lastly, very few of these products are designed for use in partial hand amputation.

Task specific prosthesis are beneficial for patients with specialized vocational or recreational needs (that is, hooks for wires/cables etc., hammer and saw attachments, components to allow a prop for rifle or archery shooting, or playing a musical instrument, to name a few). This may require extending the socket onto the forearm to allow for effective counterbalance when lifting heavy objects. Various quick connect/disconnect devices are available to allow for efficient use of multiple terminal devices with a single socket. It should be kept in mind, however, that sockets made to accommodate heavier loads can often interfere with effective wrist motion; as such, the patient's residual strength and skin integrity should be taken into consideration.

Cosmetic covers can be engineered out of PVC, vinyl, or silicone to provide a base to an extremely life-like coating that can match the skin tone and characteristics of the intact limb. The covers can also be textured to increase grip and to decrease friction against clothing and material. These covers, however, are not as durable as exposed metal or thermoplastic terminal devices and are not designed for heavy use. Often a more durable cover can be fabricated for use during more demanding tasks and the patient can change the covers as the situation dictates.

Prosthetic Options for Partial Hand Amputees

Non-Functional Passive Prosthesis

A non-functional passive prosthesis for an amputee with partial hand amputation typically consists of a cosmetic glove (made of PVC, vinyl, or silicone) filled with urethane foam with or without wire reinforcements running the length to provide stability and help resist deformation. For amputees with digit loss that does not require a full glove, individual digits can be fabricated. One of the primary challenges of this type of prosthesis is suspension. It is most typically provided by adhesive coatings or adhesive tapes and these can be more or less effective depending on body chemistry, perspiration, and how the prosthesis is used. The covering materials each have inherent advantages and disadvantages. Polyvinyl chloride is durable to mechanical stresses and is relatively inexpensive; however it tends to degrade over time. This degradation process can increase with frequent exposure to sunlight. PVC coverings also tend to pick up environmental contaminants, such as newspaper print, more easily. They are typically manufactured in a range of skin tones but exact matching and contouring to the patient's intact hand are not routinely done with this material. Silicone is a more robust material. When cured, it will retain its original shape and mechanical properties even when exposed to heat (similar to silicone bakeware) and environmental contaminants. Though silicone will not degrade in sunlight, it does tend to fade and the caliber of the material used for cosmetic covers tends to tear easily. In non-functional passive prosthesis the silicone can be thicker and more wear and tear resistant, but when covering functional units, the silicone must be thin enough to allow for range of motion and to not create any significant resistance to movement. Lastly, high grade silicones, especially if they are highly customized, can be very expensive. Customization can include the creation of an exact mirror image of the intact hand including vein patterns, skin imperfections/discolorations, and nail beds.

Functional Passive or "Static" Prosthesis

Functional passive or "static" prostheses are typically very task specific, and usually are used for a specific purpose and then removed. They have no moving parts and often function simply as an oppositional or axial loading buttress. These may be especially useful in amputees who have a functioning thumb but no other digits present to perform a functional oppositional grip. The majority of prostheses in this category bear little resemblance to a natural hand. These devices are especially suited for task specific needs such as handling tools or cooking utensils and it is helpful for the patient to bring the object that will be used, so that a specific prosthesis can be fabricated to meet those needs. For rugged applications such as factory work or heavy labor, these are usually made of stainless steel and shaped to meet the needs of the amputee. If needed or desired, a skin-tone colored Plastisol (plastic) cover can be added to increase friction for gripping. For less demanding work but the continued need for a more complete hand structure, Plastisol can be laminated over a shaped wood such as lightweight balsa or aluminum covered with polyurethane foam. Light thermoplastics can also be used and can be fabricated in almost any shape.

Active Body-Powered Prostheses

Active body-powered prostheses for patients with partial hand amputation can be finger, wrist or shoulder driven. Finger driven devices use the intrinsic muscles of the hand and require the use of at least one intact metacarpophalangeal joint. Shoulder driven devices are powered by biscapular abduction and/or glenohumeral flexion and wrist powered by flexion or extension of that joint. A figure-of-nine harness must be worn if shoulder power is used. This can be restrictive and it requires abnormal movements of the shoulders to activate the terminal device, most commonly a voluntary opening hook or claw. A couple of the more common cable-powered devices for partial hand amputees, the Handy Hook/Handy Wrist combination and the Robin Aids hand are no longer commercially available but may still be encountered in the clinical setting. Both of these were manufactured by the United States Manufacturing Company, Pasadena, CA, that now produces the newer version of the Robin Aids hand, which, though not designed for partial hand amputee use, can be modified for that purpose by a skilled prosthetist. Wrist flexion/extension devices operate in a similar manner of the tenodesis grip hand orthosis. Tenodesis is a functional action that entails creating prehension using the thumb and the index finger and/or the middle finger by flexing the wrist. This prosthesis depends on the amputee's strength and range of motion at the wrist to create closing (wrist flexion) and opening of the digits (wrist extension). The greatest limitation of the tenodesis prosthesis using wrist flexion/extension is that it greatly restricts freely positioning the hand in space, limiting its functional utility. A prosthesis that allows free wrist motion to be maintained greatly increases overall hand function. This is where powered prosthesis can greatly improve the dynamic cosmesis (how natural a device appears when in motion/use) of a partial hand prosthesis.

Externally Powered Devices

Externally powered devices for the partial hand amputee can be advantageous for many reasons. They are entirely self-contained which makes donning and doffing the device much easier. They do not require restrictive suspension or cabling across the wrist, arm, or elbow thereby decreasing the potential for skin irritation especially in patients who may have scar tissue and/or hypersensitivity. Also, these devices eliminate the need for significant wrist range of motion for force generation. A distinct disadvantage of all externally powered devices is the loss of proprioception inherent to cable driven systems. Also, due to the length of the residual limb, adding a self-contained prosthetic unit can be aesthetically displeasing to the amputee because it could be longer than the sound limb. Only a few prosthetic companies currently manufacture purpose built partial hand units but many units can be modified or purpose built by a skilled prosthetist to meet the needs of a partial hand amputee and more specifically the short transmetacarpal amputee (see the section on advanced technologies). Suspension includes a custom molded socket that encompasses the dorsum of the hand with an effort to leave the palm exposed for sensory input and the wrist minimally encumbered for free function. A flexible silicone sleeve that extends above the wrist can be added to increase suction and leverage. The terminal device can be anything from a simple two pronged hook device or claw device to individually control finger units. The functional motions are generated using myoelectric interfaces firmly pressed against functioning, and typically antagonistic, proximal muscle pairs. As with most myoelectric interfaces, motion can be activated by a single contraction signal, by a series of contraction signals at the same muscle, by controlled co-contraction of muscle pairs, or by proportional control. The coordination of these muscle actions takes time and effort but for a motivated amputee can allow for a very functional powered prosthetic unit.

To decrease the complexity of movement as more functional components (motors) are added, some companies are developing terminal devices that operate using synergistic motion patterns. For example, a muscle contraction signal that operates one motor unit at a pre-programmed force and speed will also activate one or more other motor units at variable pre-programmed forces/speeds. Functionally this could be used to create more force than speed at the prosthetic thumb unit and more speed than force at the opposite prosthetic prehensile unit (either a single unit or a combination of units) to create a motion and grip pattern that is more natural than all units moving at the same speed and generating the same force.

The vast majority of innovation and advances in micromechanics and microprocessors for current prosthetic devices occur in the externally powered category. Motors and servos that drive the articulating interfaces of these devices are becoming smaller, lighter, and more efficient. This allows more human-like motion and, along with more flexible and durable cosmetic covers, natural appearance of the prosthesis. That said, technology is expensive and often not covered by insurances. Many if not most amputees with partial hand amputation can find acceptable function with the use of very basic passive, passive functional, or body-powered prostheses. Their inherent advantages of being lighter in weight, typically less bulky, fewer or no moving parts, requiring much less maintenance (lay and expert), and reasonable cost will ensure that, regardless of technological advances, these prostheses will continue to be used.

Advanced Technologies for Partial Hand and Transmetacarpal Amputees

Robotic prosthetic hands with individually articulating fingers, though often cost prohibitive, are currently available on the retail market. When originally introduced, these hands were revolutionary in their appearance and function and shattered the accepted aesthetic of available hand prostheses at the time. Touch Bionics was the first to introduce a product in this category when it manufactured the "I-limb" (Figure 14.2). With these devices, each finger contains its own motor and gearbox. This hand can be modified to accommodate partial hand amputees. The I-digit is also available when individual (but usually two or more) fingers are missing. Input is controlled through myoelectric sensors that read signals from muscles that would normally be used to activate an intact hand. The I-limb does not have a powered thumb. It can be manually positioned to allow for a key (lateral) or cylindrical grasp pattern and is held in place by friction. The "BeBionic" hand by RSLSteeper is essentially identical in functional capability as the I-limb. Otto Bock has developed the "Transcarpal" hand specifically for amputees with long residual limbs, including those with transcarpal amputations. Essentially this hand provides a self-contained small volume hand unit with the thumb unit fixed in adduction in order to provide a highly functional three-jaw chuck grip pattern against two finger extensions that move simultaneously on the same actuator.

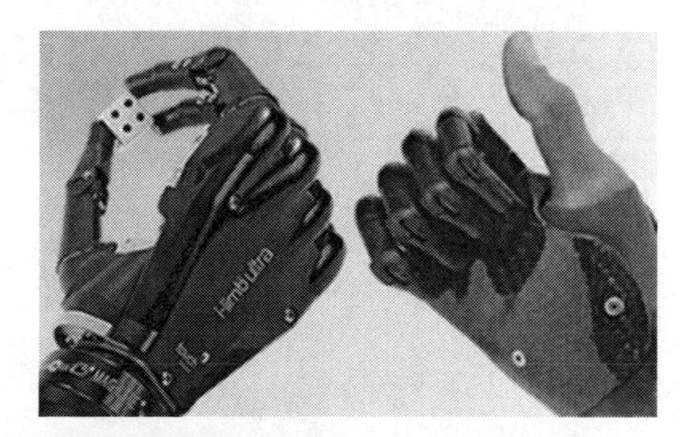

Figure 14.2 I-limb and I-digits.
***Source*: From Touch Bionics, Mansfield, MA. Used with permission.**

REFERENCES

1. Dillingham T, MacKenzie E. Limb amputation and limb deficiency: Epidemiology and recent trends in the United States. *South Med J.* 2002 Aug;95(8):875–883.
2. Wedderburn, Caldwell, Sanderson, Olive. A wrist-powered prosthesis for the partial hand. *JACPOC.* 1986;21(3):42.
3. Cuccurullo S. *Physical Medicine and Rehabilitation Board Review*. Demos Medical Publishing; 2004.
4. Roeschlein RA, Domholdt E. Factors related to successful upper extremity prosthetic use. *Prosthet Orthot Int*. 1989;13:14–18.
5. Fraser CM. An evaluation of the use made of cosmetic and functional prostheses by unilateral upper limb amputees. *Prosthet Orthot Int*. 1998;22:216–223.

15

Prosthetic Prescriptions for Long Transradial Amputations

Christopher Fantini

The purpose of this chapter is to provide the reader with a general background and review of upper extremity (UE) prosthetic principles and provide discussion on those of long transradial (TR) amputations, including wrist disarticulations (WDs). Brief descriptions of the surgical procedures, fitting concepts and prosthetic designs, are included to better inform the reader of prescription rationale. However, a detailed discussion of these topics lies beyond the scope of this chapter. The reader should refer to the publications cited in the references, as well as the additional resources located at the end of the chapter, for further information.

WHY CONSIDER UPPER EXTREMITY PROSTHESES?

Upper limb amputations are predominantly caused by trauma [1–3]. It is currently impossible to replace all of the lost functions secondary to the amputation of any part of the hand or arm as the human upper limb is extremely complex.

The shoulder complex, elbow, wrist and hand, together, create a field of movement that can be referred to as the "functional envelope" (see example in Figure 15.1). This envelope, composed of several integrated arcs of movement, is determined by the degrees of freedom (DOF) and range of motion (ROM) at each joint [4].

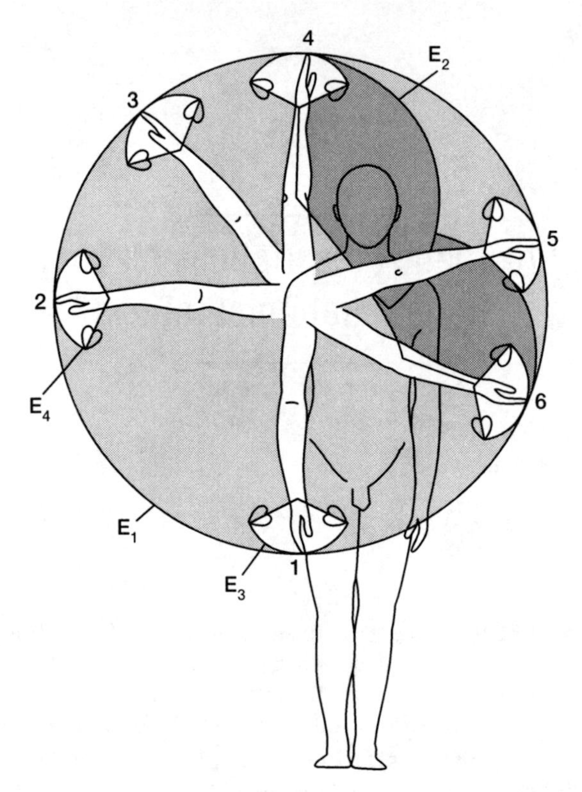

Figure 15.1 Some of the ROM constituting the functional envelope in the intact upper limb.
***Source*: Adapted from [12].**

One DOF is equivalent to a single axis of motion. For example, the axis for wrist flexion and extension constitutes a single DOF in the wrist, while the axis for radial/ulnar deviation constitutes a second DOF. Limitation, or absence as with an amputation, in the active range of motion (AROM), or DOF, in any joint, will limit the functional capacity of the upper limb by reducing the effective size of the "envelope." Any task, requiring the need to reach a point outside of the functional envelope, requires compensatory strategies in the remnant limb, trunk, and/or lower limbs. Depending on the degree of difficulty with compensating for the lost ROM, an individual may avoid certain functional tasks altogether. Other tasks, which cannot be avoided, may require compensatory strategies that, when repeated enough over time, can cause injuries resulting from poor posture or overuse syndromes [5,6].

Though no single prosthesis can replace all lost functions, individuals with UE limb deficiencies do have several prosthetic options available, which can facilitate some functional recovery and may reduce the likelihood of potential injury from compensatory motion or overuse syndromes in the sound limb. The types of options considered depends on factors such as the following:

- Amputation level
- Patient's goals/motivation
- Patient's living conditions/support
- Patient's cognitive abilities
- Access to appropriate health care (a team experienced with UE prosthetics and rehabilitation)
- Patient's financial coverage/resource

Individuals with amputation at the TR level, tend to utilize prostheses at a higher rate than those with amputations at other levels [7,8]. Prosthetic options for individuals with upper limb amputations, with special attention toward long TR residuums (those with 50%–100% of the radius/ulna remaining) (example seen in Figure 15.2), including those with WD, will be discussed in this text.

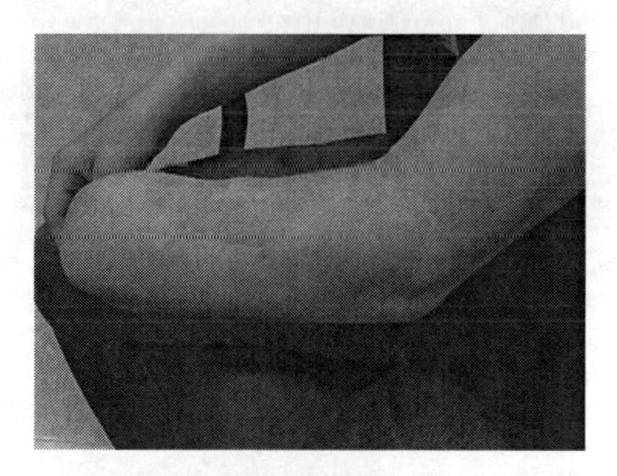

Figure 15.2 A long, left, TR residual limb.

SURGICAL TECHNIQUES

The surgical technique used in the amputation process has a significant impact on the style and control scheme of any potential prosthesis. The following are surgical procedures which can be utilized at the TR level.

- Myoplasty – The suturing of agonist–antagonist muscle pairs to each other.
- Myodesis – Direct suturing of residual limb musculature or tendon to bone/periosteum.
- Cineplasty – Surgical isolation of a loop of muscle, covering it with skin, and attaching it to a terminal device (TD) to be operated by contraction of the muscle in the loop. This is not a very common procedure but it is usually done with the biceps or pectoral musculature (see Figure 15.3).

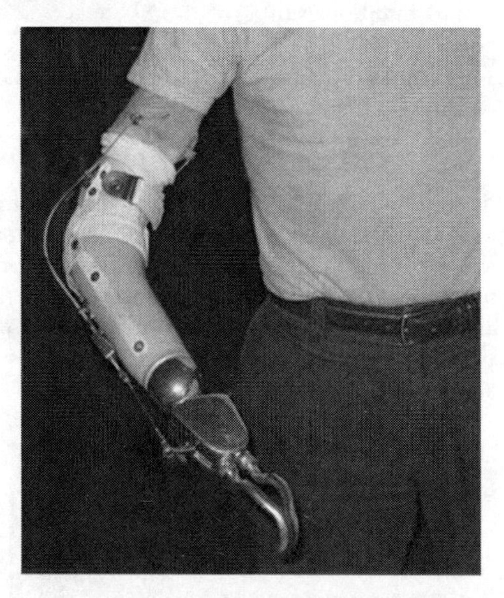

Figure 15.3 Biceps cineplasty prosthesis—the wearer applies tension to the control cable, by utilizing a biceps contraction, to voluntarily close the hook.

- Krukenberg – Separation of the radius/ulna is best indicated for blind, bilateral TR amputees because it preserves tactile function and provides the individual the ability to reach and grasp objects.
- Osseointegration – Direct skeletal attachment of the prosthesis via a titanium abutment, which protrudes through the skin from the cut end of the bone [9].

Most amputation surgeries at the TR level involve a combination of myodesis, with the deeper layers of the forearm musculature, and myoplasty, with the more superficial ones. Traditionally, the dominant principle in amputation surgery has been to save as much length of the limb as possible. When discussing TR amputations, the anatomical

ROM for pronation/supination remaining after surgery is proportionally related to the length of the remaining forearm (see Figure 15.4).

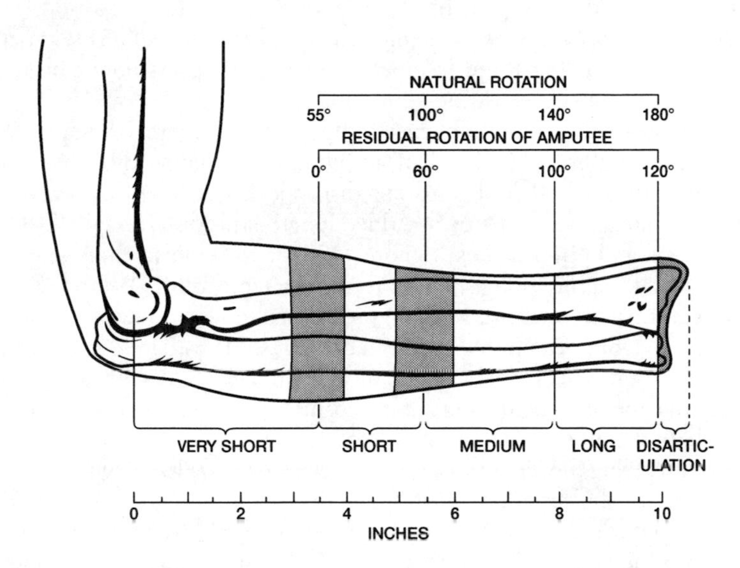

Figure 15.4 Transradial amputation lengths and corresponding potential for pronation/supination.
***Source*: Adapted from [13].**

Wrist disarticulations preserve the maximum length of the forearm and can provide the patient with several advantages for using a prosthesis (see Table 15.1). These include the potential of full ROM for voluntary pronation/supination, maximum forearm leverage, and use of the distal styloids of the radius and ulna for suspension of the prosthetic device.

However, amputation at this level does not always result in the most functional prosthetic outcome. If, for any reason, the surgery is not expected to preserve a significant range of anatomical pronation/supination and/or the patient's soft tissue is not expected to tolerate the suspension forces over the styloids of the radius and ulna, then an amputation at the TR level would serve them better. Even when WDs do provide the advantages previously listed, they result in very limited options with choosing prosthetic components and, in the unilateral case, commonly result in a length discrepancy, between the prosthesis and the sound limb, which is often aesthetically unacceptable to the patient.

Alternatively, those with unilateral, long TR residual limbs usually have the advantage of maintaining a significant level of anatomical pronation and supination (as opposed to amputations resulting in shorter residuums), and provide the patient and prosthetist a much broader selection of prosthetic components to choose from (for example, the option of using an electric, quick disconnect [QD], wrist unit that allows the patient to change powered TDs) without causing a length discrepancy with the sound limb.

In bilateral upper limb cases, the prostheses can be made to matching lengths at any level of amputation, including those with a WD on either or both limbs. Adding disproportionate length, however, is not advantageous to the user. Added length adds distal weight to the prosthesis and often makes it more difficult to perform functions at midline (such as fastening shirt buttons or bringing the TD of the prosthesis toward the mouth). Making prostheses too long may also result in the need for the amputee to purchase new shirts with longer sleeves, adding expense. It is ideal to keep all UE prostheses as short as possible, while maintaining the amputee's cosmetic concerns, to transfer the weight of the prosthesis more proximally and facilitate the ability of the wearer to bring the TD to midline for activities of daily living (ADL).

Due to the fact that most upper limb amputations are caused by trauma, it is not always possible for the patient, doctor, surgeon, and prosthetist to collaborate on surgical considerations for a specific case. Surgeons and doctors who deal with upper limb amputees should maintain a regular, open, line of communication with a prosthetist experienced in fitting this population, so that general concepts and advancements in prosthetic fitting procedures can be shared. Whenever possible, prior to surgery, the patient should be made aware of the pros and cons of undergoing a WD procedure versus a long TR amputation, so that the best decision can be made. This will maximize the patient's functional recovery and quality of life.

Table 15.1 Wrist Disarticulation Amputation: Considerations for a Prosthesis

Pros	Cons
Potential of full ROM for anatomical pronation/supination	Commonly results in length discrepancy between the prosthesis and sound limb (however this is not a factor for the bilateral UE amputee)
Provides maximum forearm leverage	
Allows suspension of the prosthesis over the distal styloids of the radius and ulna	Significantly limits choices in selecting prosthetic components

The prescription of a TR prosthesis requires decisions in the selection of its major features. The overall design/control option and the specific features of the prosthesis itself, which include the interface/socket design, suspension method, wrist unit, and TD, need to be determined according to the patient's goals.

PROSTHETIC OPTIONS

Individuals faced with amputation should be fully informed of all available options and empowered to be the primary driver in the decision-making process to maximize positive outcomes. All individuals who have undergone UE amputation have the following six options relating to prosthetic devices (as well as combinations thereof): No prosthesis; Semi-Prehensile Cosmetic Prosthesis; Body Powered Cable-Driven Prosthesis; Externally Powered Prosthesis; Hybrid Prosthesis; and Specialty Prosthesis. A brief discussion of each option follows:

No Prosthesis

A person may decide not to wear a prosthesis for many reasons, such as the following:

- They're unaware of their options
- Had a bad experience with previously trying a prosthesis
- Body image issues
- Their efficiency of being "one-handed"
- Limited functional ability of current technology
- Financial limitations
- Lack of skilled prosthetic training
- Semi-prehensile cosmetic design
- Body powered (cable-driven) design
- Externally powered design
- Hybrid design
- Specialty/task specific design

A brief list of the pros and cons of this option can be seen in Table 15.2.

Semi-Prehensile Cosmetic Prosthesis

This prosthetic option uses materials such as polyvinyl chloride (PVC), micro-coated vinyl (MCV) or silicone, to produce a prosthesis meant to maximize cosmetic appeal but there are other functional benefits, beyond

Table 15.2 Pros and Cons of Choosing Not to Use a Prosthesis

Pros	Cons
Simplicity	Poor aesthetics
Comfort – no harness or sockets	Smallest functional envelope of the six options
Sensation – residuum is not encapsulated, thereby allowing full sensory feedback with external environment	Necessitates either functioning as "one-handed" or "no-hands," in the case of bilaterals
Improved mobility as compared to wearing a prosthesis	Reduced ability for bimanual tasks

aesthetics. It can provide practical function, as it facilitates bimanual tasks (such as carrying large objects) and the semi-prehensile fingers can be positioned for function in specific activities, such as grabbing handles and holding utensils or other small object and tools (see Figure 15.5).

PVC is cheaper than its silicone alternative but stains much more easily and typically needs replacement after a few months. MCV gloves are more cosmetic and resistant to stains than PVC gloves but are more expensive (see Figures 15.5 and 15.6). In comparison, a custom silicone prosthesis offers the most lifelike appearance, is more durable (can last for years when properly maintained) and has excellent resistance to staining (see Figure 15.6). It is, however, significantly more expensive and does not afford the same functional capacity as the body

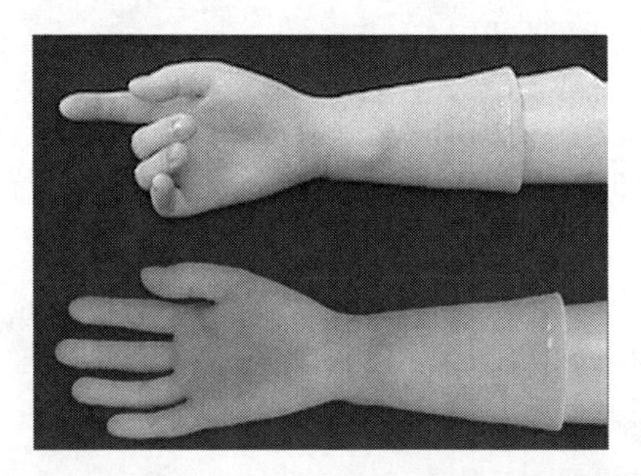

Figure 15.5 Prefabricated semi-prehensile MCV cosmetic hand in an open position and a finger point position, which can be useful for typing or pushing buttons.

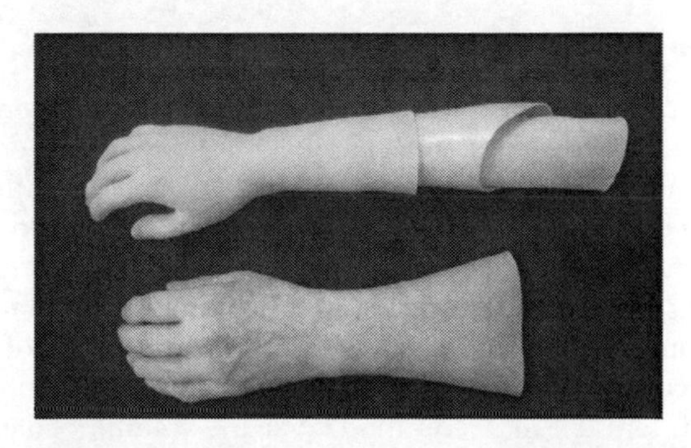

Figure 15.6 The top prosthesis is the same semi-prehensile prosthesis shown in Figure 15.5, with an MCV-covered hand. The bottom prosthesis is a custom silicone design showing more lifelike appearance and detail.

powered, externally powered, or hybrid designs. A brief summary of the pros and cons of this option can be seen in Table 15.3.

Table 15.3 Pros and Cons of a Semi-Prehensile Cosmetic Prosthesis

Pros	Cons
Cosmetic appearance can be made very lifelike with silicone, which resists stains	PVC products (a type of material used to make non-custom cosmetic gloves) easily stain
No harnessing necessary for TR level. Only minimal harnessing may be needed for higher levels of amputation	May require topical agents for donning and suspension
	Custom silicone devices are expensive
Relatively lightweight and inexpensive	No active control of the fingers (they have to be positioned and manipulated by external forces)
Can have semi-prehensile, flexible fingers which can be prepositioned for specific functions or to hold specific objects	
Can accommodate any level of amputation without causing a length discrepancy with the sound limb	

Body Powered Cable-Driven Prosthesis

This type of prosthesis utilizes straps and cables to control the motions of the prosthesis. This can be an effective prescription for a new amputee, in early post-op fitting. Although any other option could be considered if appropriate, the body powered design is inexpensive and functional. There are also therapeutic rationale for considering the body powered system for a new amputee: it helps improve joint ROM through active control of the TD; desensitizes the limb; controls edema as it shapes the limb for a more definitive socket; and it can accommodate shape/volume changes in the residual limb, as the healing process progresses, with the addition of socks (which minimizes the frequency of required interface/socket replacements). A list of the pros and cons are seen in Table 15.4.

Table 15.4 Pros and Cons of a Body Powered Prosthesis

Pros	Cons
Greater functional capacity than semi-prehensile devices	Requires harnessing, which can compromise comfort and restrict movement
Durable, can be used for heavy duty activities and harsh environments (water, dirt, etc.)	Requires a certain level of strength and ROM in the residuum
Provides proprioceptive feedback through the harness and socket	Decreased grip force as compared to externally powered TDs
Faster response than externally powered devices	May lack the cosmetic appeal of semi-prehensile or powered devices
Less expensive than externally powered devices	Axillary pressure from harness may lead to nerve entrapment syndrome over time
Lower maintenance costs—no battery required	

Externally Powered Prosthesis

Externally powered prostheses use battery power, control inputs, and actuators to control motion and grip force in a prosthesis. These devices should only be fit on a mature residual limb, that is, one stable in volume. Generally, the externally powered prosthesis is fit six months, or later, post amputation. Externally powered devices are typically heavier, the most costly and require the most maintenance, among all the designs. For this reason, these devices should only be considered if certain factors are met. The potential user should have at least one good muscle signal, from their residuum, that they can be trained to use for operating an externally powered device. If other inputs are being considered, such as force sensitive resistors or linear transducers, the patient must have sufficient ROM and strength to operate the control inputs. Another factor that needs to be considered is the patient's accessibility to a prosthetics facility that has adequate experience in fitting such devices. In addition, the funding source needs to be considered since this device, as stated earlier, is expensive and will require routine maintenance costs as well as new replacements every 3 to 5 years. Finally, this option should only be considered if the above-mentioned factors are met and the patient understands, and is committed to, the requirements of following a functional training program with an experienced prosthetist and occupational therapist.

In the case of the WD or long TR amputee, the residual musculature is generally intact and usually provides very good antagonistic muscle signals for dual site control. Dual site EMG (muscle) control simply means that the amputee exhibits good EMG signal separation for two independent, antagonistic muscle signals, in this case, the forearm flexors and the extensors. A summary of the pros and cons of this design option is listed in Table 15.5.

Hybrid Design for Amputation Levels at or Above the Elbow

The hybrid design combines the use of body powered and externally powered components in a single prosthesis. Though possible for the shorter transradial limb, this option is not considered for a WD, and would be extremely unusual for a long TR level, prosthesis. It is most often used with transhumeral and shoulder level prostheses (see corresponding chapters for more discussion).

Specialty/Adaptive Design

When an individual with UE limb loss wishes to continue, or begin, an activity or hobby that cannot be adequately accommodated with the previously described options, the use of a specialty prosthesis may be considered. These devices can be made for specific vocational tasks, such as holding particular tools, but are generally made for recreational/sporting activities such as swimming, cycling, weight lifting, golf, playing a musical instrument, etc. (see Figures 15.7 and 15.8). Table 15.7 provides a brief summary of the pros and cons of using specialty/adaptive prostheses.

Table 15.5 Pros and Cons of an Externally Powered Prosthesis

Pros	Cons
Eliminates/minimizes the need for harnessing	Much more expensive to purchase and maintain (more susceptible to damage from moisture and vibration/impact)
Electric TDs* have increased grip force as compared to body powered ones	Generally used for light duty activities only and basic ADLs. Not intended for heavy duty workload
More natural control through use of residual muscles, especially for proportional control	Lack of proprioception in relation to TD position and open/close state as compared to harness design
Increased functional envelope—due to ability to use device in all planes of arm movement, easier wrist control and increased TD function (especially with multi-articulated hands)	Increased weight
	Must be charged on a regular basis
	Must have excellent socket fit to maintain function. Weight or limb volume fluctuations will have a negative impact on function when using EMG electrodes
Improved aesthetics as compared to body powered design	Excessive perspiration can also adversely affect EMG control signal
Some multi-articulated, externally powered prosthetic hands allow specific grip patterns to be programmed into the device and selected, on command, by the user	Limited powered motions—only a maximum of four effective powered DOF are currently commercially available (hand open/close; isolated thumb flexion/extension; wrist pronation/supination; and elbow flexion/extension)

*TD = "terminal device"—term used to describe the most distal aspect of the prosthesis which is designed to perform grasping or some other specific function. It is usually a prosthetic hand or hook but can be a specialty tool.

Some individuals may use more than one of the options listed above. For example, they may have a body powered prosthesis they use for yard work, an externally powered, myoelectrically controlled prosthesis they use for their office job and a specialty prosthesis used for fishing. In addition to the rationale implied in this example, that is, using a specific prosthesis in particular

Table 15.6 Pros and Cons of a Hybrid Prosthesis

Pros	Cons
Larger functional envelope than body powered system	Harness is needed for body powered function (usually elbow control)
Less expensive than devices that are completely externally powered	For shorter limbs, more demand on strength and residuum ROM to get full ROM in the prosthetic joint
Lower weight than externally powered	Potential for more maintenance
Stronger grip force available as compared with body powered devices	

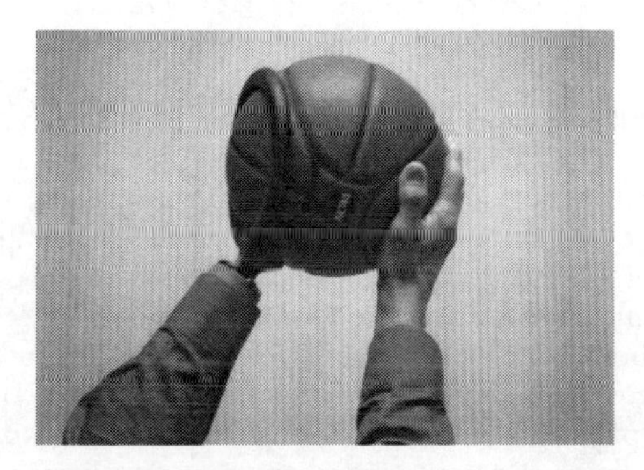

Figure 15.7 Basketball-inspired TD.

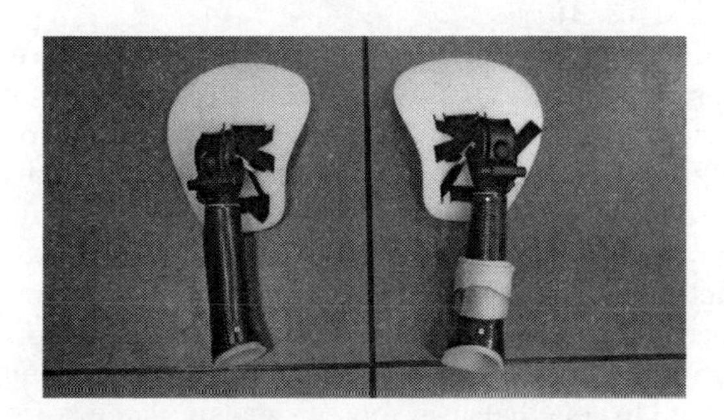

Figure 15.8 Bilateral prostheses, self-suspending, with paddles for kayaking/canoeing.

Table 15.7 Pros and Cons of a Specialty/Adaptive Prosthesis

Pros	Cons
Customized for a specific function/task Can empower the individual to return to participating in the same recreational activities as before the amputation	Limited function outside of its intended purpose

settings for different functions, it should be strongly advocated that all users of UE prostheses get at least two prosthetic devices, even if they are both of the same design. The reason is that every prosthesis, at some point, will need maintenance or breakdown, especially in regard to the more active, rugged, wearers. In some cases, the need may be very simple, enabling the amputee to perform the repair themselves, with some spare parts, eliminating the need for a visit to the prosthetist's office. Other issues may require a visit to the prosthetist but can be repaired that same day, while the patient waits. Still, other problems, such as catastrophic component or material failure, may require complete overhauls to the interface or components, possibly leaving the amputee without the device for days or even weeks. Given these possibilities, it is essential that each amputee has at least one functional alternative to their primary prosthesis to ensure continued function and quality of life, should such repairs be needed. In line with this philosophy, the Department of Defense military hospitals currently provide each service member, requiring upper limb prostheses, multiple prosthetic devices, often three or more, usually of different designs [10].

The design and fitting of the alternative prosthesis(es) should begin after a satisfactory result has been achieved with that of the initial device. This will minimize the need for multiple fittings of the interface of each subsequent prosthesis, should the same interface style be used, and will have provided the amputee the opportunity to gain some experience with using a prosthesis, giving them a better perspective as to what they may want in an alternate device. This approach facilitates a more appropriate, cost effective, method for achieving the individual's personal goals. It is important to note that an amputee's goals and needs are not fixed variables, but can, and often do, change over time. Developments in the individual's physical condition, social status, vocation, and/or technological advancements in prosthetic components, can influence changes in the individual's fitting needs and goals. Achieving these new goals may require changes to the design of existing prosthesis(es), or warrant the prescription of a completely new one.

ANATOMY OF THE PROSTHESIS

A prosthesis is made up of a combination of components. At the WD and long TR level, they can be summarized in the following categories:

- Prosthetic interface (socket)
- Suspension method
- Wrist unit
- Terminal device

Prosthetic Interface

The term "interface" is used throughout Chapters 15–17 to better describe what is traditionally called the "socket." Other contributors to this text may use the term "socket" within their description of the prosthesis. This author uses the terms interchangeably but agrees with those who favor the term "interface," as it better reflects the advancements in materials and fitting designs than does the former term "socket," which denotes a simple "plug-in" concept.

The prosthetic interface, or socket, refers to the component of the prosthesis that is in closest contact with the residuum. The prosthetic interface can be made of a flexible thermoplastic material, to provide total contact with the limb, surrounded by a rigid frame which keeps pressure over tolerant areas (Figure 15.9). The interface may also be in the form of a silicone or gel liner which rolls onto the limb and is then inserted into the rigid frame and held in place with a pin locking or lanyard system (Figure 15.10). Lanyard systems are more appropriate for use with the long TR limb, should this type of suspension be used, as the pin locking systems add too much length to the prosthesis due to the required locking mechanism needed.

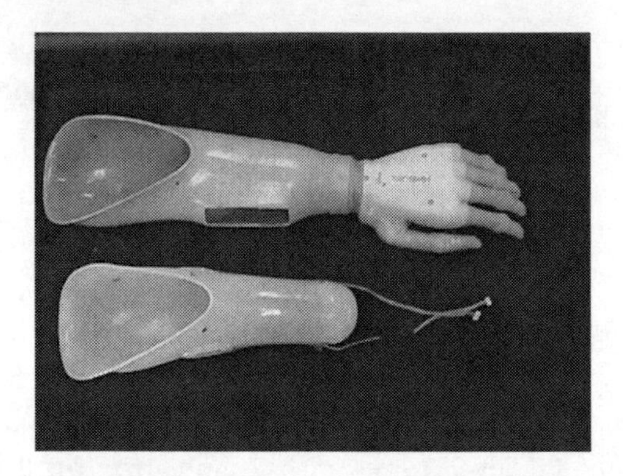

Figure 15.9 A left myoelectric, Northwestern style, self-suspending prosthesis for a long TR limb. The thermoflexible socket has been removed from the rigid laminated frame. The wires for the electrodes are shown and connect to the inner surface of the wrist unit for operation of the TD.

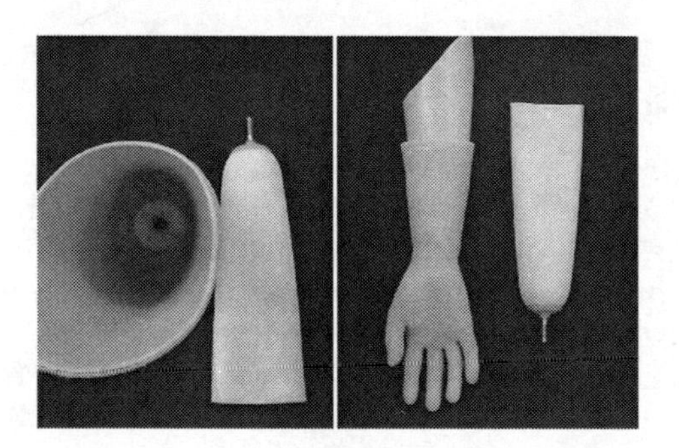

Figure 15.10 A right, self-suspended, semi-prehensile prosthesis using a roll-on silicone locking liner as seen on the right side of the socket in each image. The liner is rolled onto the limb, and then the limb is inserted into the frame. The pin on the liner engages with the lock at the distal end of the frame, which is seen in the view of the prosthesis in the transverse plane on the left, and suspension is achieved.

Typically the interface is removable from the frame, as seen in Figures 15.9 and 15.10, but sometimes they are one and the same. The latter is commonly referred to as a "hard socket."

The design of the long TR or WD prosthetic interface is influenced by several factors including the residual limb length and the prosthetic control system being considered. The common goals of any upper limb prosthetic interface design are to maximize ROM, comfortably spread the load forces during active lift, stabilize the prosthesis against rotary forces, and support vertical loading.

The ROM is affected by limb length and interface design. As a general rule, the longer the residual limb, the more distal the trimlines (proximal edges) of the interface can be on the limb. Lower trimlines generally allow for a more voluntary ROM.

The forces on the residual limb during active lifting, when using a prosthesis, are proportional to the radial and ulnar surface areas of the interface. During lifting activities, with TR and WD prostheses, a force couple is created, which results in focused pressure on the distal radial and proximal ulnar aspects of the limb (see Figure 15.11). When the prosthesis is intended for heavy duty use, meaning larger loads will be carried, the ulnar trimline of the interface can extend up to, and even include, the olecranon to maximize the distribution of the load. (Figure 15.11 shows an example of long TR or WD trimlines and the direction of force couple during active lift.)

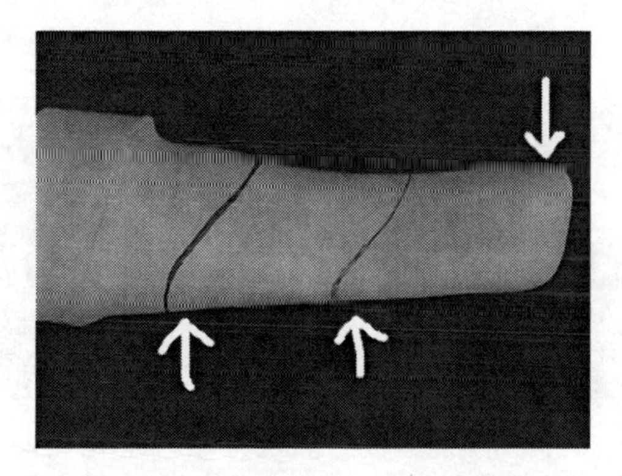

Figure 15.11 A plaster model of a left WD with two different levels of sample trimlines drawn, and arrows indicating the direction of force couple during active lift. The longer the ulnar trimline, the more the force of active lift is dispersed on the forearm.

When the residual limb is long, as with the case of a WD or long TR, the interface is made to intimately fit with the shape and contours of the distal forearm, specifically in the area of the interosseous membrane. This produces an interface shape often described as a "screwdriver fit," due to the relative flattening of shape at the distal forearm (see Figures 15.12 and 15.13), which stabilizes the prosthesis against rotary forces, such as when turning a doorknob.

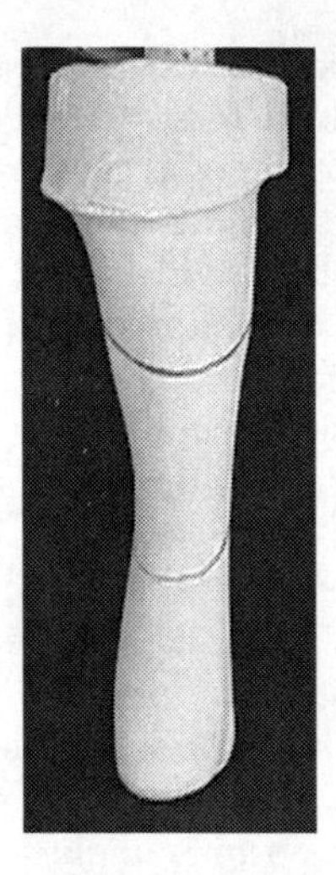

Figure 15.12 Anterior view of left WD plaster mold showing the anatomical contours that can be used for suspension and control.

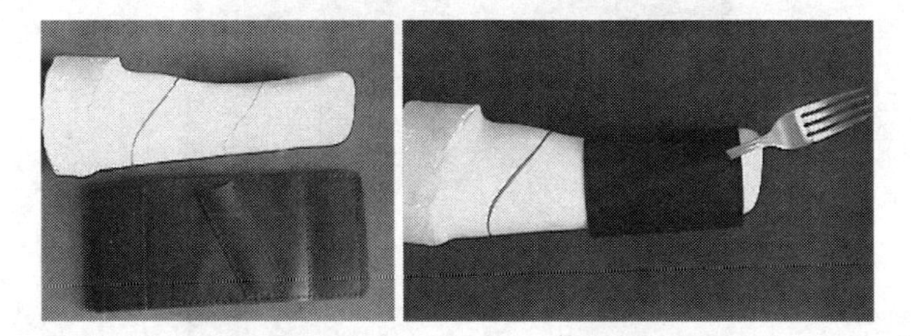

Figure 15.13 A custom leather cuff, wrapped on a plaster mold of a left WD, with a sewn pocket for holding utensils such as a fork. This cuff wraps around the forearm and attaches to itself via Velcro. This is a good alternative to have, for individuals with long TR residual limbs or WD, in addition to a prosthesis.

Other possibilities for the WD or long TR amputee include that of a simple forearm cuff featuring either a pocket or mechanical attachment mechanism, which enables the amputee to utilize utensils or hold a pen/pencil (see Figure 15.13). This option is great for individuals who do not always want to wear a prosthesis but still prefer improved function to not using a device at all. It is very inexpensive, easy to make, and versatile.

It is ideal to allow the amputee to try out different interface designs during the trial fitting period before a definitive design is selected. This trial period may last 2–3 weeks or up to several months, depending on each case.

Suspension Methods

Resistance to vertical loading is accomplished through the suspension system. The prosthesis can be suspended in two ways: with the use of a harness and/or a self-suspending interface.

Harness Suspension

This method of suspension uses a series of straps to attach the prosthesis to the wearer. The vertical loading forces are distributed over the shoulders and back. Harness-suspended interfaces are well suited for prostheses that are intended for more rugged use, meaning the wearer may carry heavier loads, using the residual limb, or expose the device to harsh environments (water/moisture, dirt, chemicals, vibration etc.), which may otherwise compromise suspension of the prosthesis or lead to frequent maintenance. One downside to using a harness is that it can limit the functional mobility of the affected limb, in getting the TD to points in space.

The standard harness used to suspend a unilateral, TR, body powered, prosthesis is the figure-of-eight design (named for its shape in the horizontal plane) (An example is shown in Figure 15.14).

Body powered designs, using harness suspension, will use some form of elbow hinges. In general, elbow hinges can be either flexible (made of webbing material, leather, or wire) or rigid (single pivot). Flexible hinges are indicated for long TR, WD, and bilateral TR amputees as they preserve as much of the existing pronation/supination as possible. Flexible hinges are also indicated for children with TR amputations so as not to limit development potential by restricting movement.

Another harness design that can be used is the chest strap and shoulder saddle design. This is a better option for those who frequently have to carry heavier loads with the prosthesis as well as those who are uncomfortable with the axillary pressure exerted by a figure-of-eight harness. The chest strap and shoulder saddle design is not a common choice for WD levels and may not be desirable for many female patients as the chest strap can cause discomfort and is visible under clothing with low neck lines.

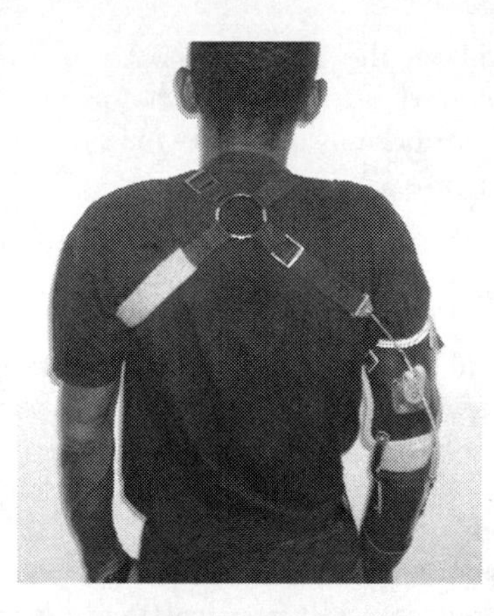

Figure 15.14 Example of a TR figure-of-eight harness design. This harness provides two functions: suspension of the prosthesis and mechanical control for the operation of the TD.

The typical body motions needed to generate the operation of a TR, or WD, cable-driven TD are biscapular abduction and/or glenohumeral flexion and abduction.

When the prosthesis, for a long TR or WD design, is suspended via a harness, the interface trimlines should be lowered to the point where at least 50% of the wearer's active pronation and supination is retained as well as 100% of available elbow flexion and extension.

All body powered, or cable-driven, systems require a harness to control the TD. However, not all cable-driven systems are suspended by a harness. They can be self-suspended.

Self-Suspension

Self-suspending interface designs eliminate the need for harnessing to suspend the prosthesis. The self-suspending interface can be held onto the residual limb by either using contours designed over bony anatomy (such as the distal styloids of the radius and ulna or the epicondyles of the humerus; see Figure 15.9) or by creating a suction environment between the limb and interface (via an intimate fit with a one-way air expulsion valve incorporated into the interface, or using silicone/gel roll-on liners or sleeves as shown in Figure 15.10). Self-suspension is often used for lighter duty prostheses such as with

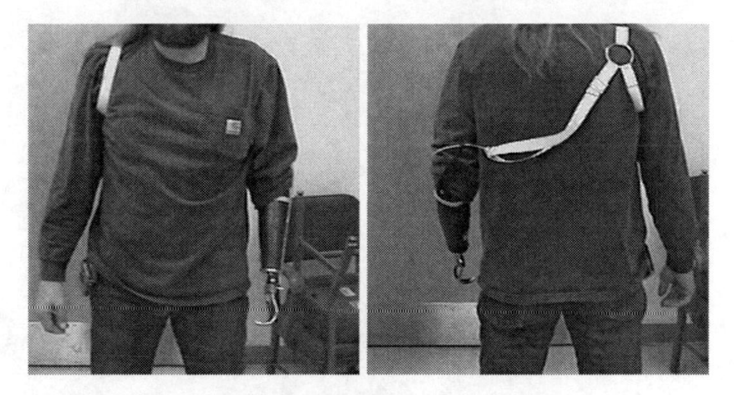

Figure 15.15 Transradial figure-of-nine harness. This is utilized for body powered TD function while using a self-suspending socket design—in this case, a silicone locking liner (hidden from view inside the interface).

externally powered and semi-prehensile cosmetic designs. They can also be used for cable-driven (with a figure-of-nine harness for TD control, as seen in Figure 15.15) designs, particularly with longer residual limbs. Usually, the long TR and WD amputee dons the prosthesis by pushing the limb into the interface.

In the case of WD, the distal styloids of the radius and ulna can provide a bony platform for suspension (suprastyloid suspension) and eliminate the need for a harness for the purpose of suspension.

The traditional self-suspending socket design for longer TR residual limbs is the Northwestern supracondylar socket design, which uses medial/lateral compression proximal to the epicondyles of the elbow (supracondylar suspension). Another supracondylar design for long TRs is called the floating brim design, where the supracondylar brim is attached to the frame of the socket via flexible strapping, similar to the flexible hinges in a TR harness. The difference is that there are no straps going over the shoulder or back. All of the resistance to distractive forces is relayed to the condyles via the attached brim. A figure-of-nine harness, however, would still be required for TD control, with any self-suspending design, should the prosthesis be cable-driven.

Self-suspending designs that encompass the olecranon can be modified for greater comfort and improved ROM by cutting a window out over the olecranon and epicondyles.

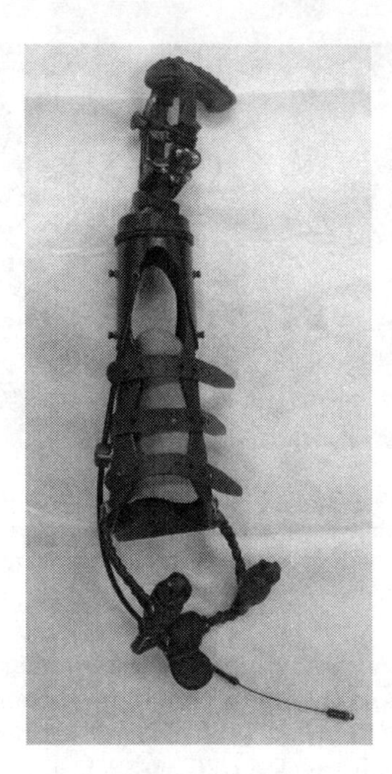

Figure 15.16 International Transradial Adjustable Limb (ITAL) made by Toughware Prosthetics Inc. (www.toughwareprx.com).

There is an option for a low cost, prefabricated, unilateral, TR prosthesis. The device is called the International Adjustable Transradial Limb (ITAL) (see Figure 15.16). It is a self-suspended, body powered prosthesis, using a supracondylar frame that attaches to the socket via flexible hinges. This device is designed for the economically challenged regions of the world and those who may live in remote areas, far from any clinical resources. However, they can be considered for amputees, in developed countries, who may have limited funding sources. They are made to be very durable and designed to allow the user to make needed repairs with simple tools and commonly available hardware supplies.

Osseointegration, in rare cases, has also been used with the TR population, with separate abutments implanted in the radius and ulna [11].

Wrist Units

The anatomical wrist has three DOF – flexion/extension, pronation/supination, and radial/ulnar deviation. As previously discussed, WD and long TR amputations can preserve all or some of the voluntary pronation/supination motion but eliminates all of the other possible movements. Prosthetic wrist units are designed to replace some of that lost function as well as to provide an attachment point for the TD.

The wrist units applicable for use with the WD or long TR should be low profile, meaning they add as little length as possible. Oval shaped wrists are available to match the shape of the distal forearm. Oval shaped wrists are better suited for prosthetic hands at this level due to the matching shape. Some common wrist units include the following:

- Standard friction wrists provide passive wrist rotation; use friction to control rotation (Figure 15.17).

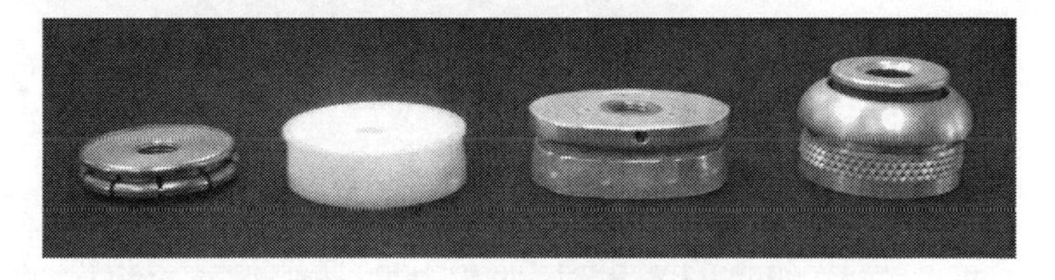

Figure 15.17 Friction wrist units—the shorter wrist units better accommodate long residual limbs in matching sound side limb lengths.

- Quick disconnect (QD), locking wrists made for both externally powered and non-powered prostheses, allow quick changing of TDs and locks in the position of the TD during grasping and lifting. The TD threads into a collar, which locks into the wrist unit chassis. These devices are not used with WD amputations. These wrist units may also create length discrepancies with the sound limb when used on certain "long" TR residuums, depending on the limb's actual length (Figure 15.18).

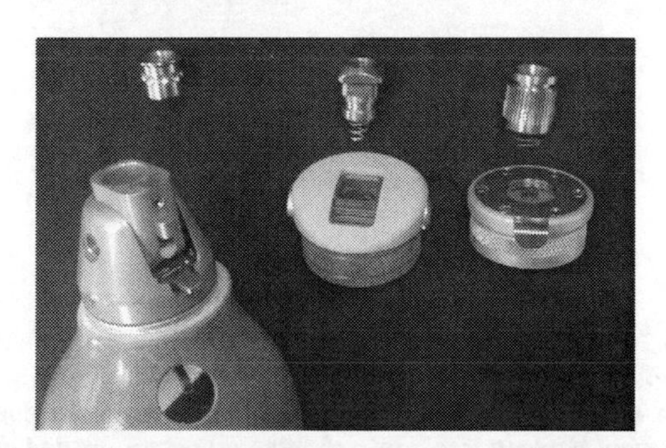

Figure 15.18 Sample of QD wrist units used for body powered TDs, with their corresponding threaded collars. A quick release button allows the collar to pop out.

- Wrist flexion units allows up to three locking positions in flexion and extension for positioning of the TD (Figure 15.19).

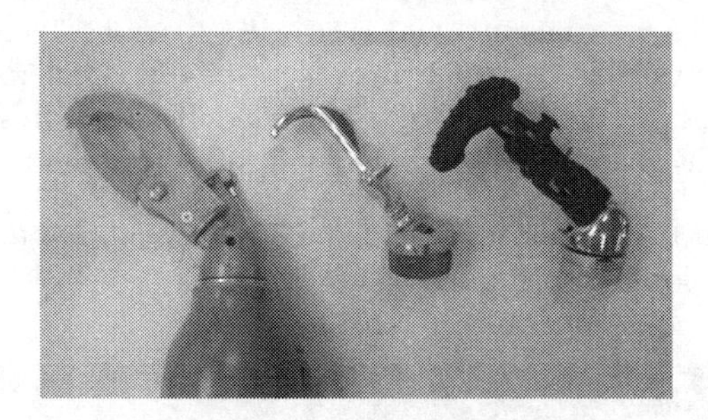

Figure 15.19 Sample wrist flexion units. All three shown also have a QD feature but this is not true of all wrist flexion units.

- Ball and socket wrists allow passive, multidirectional wrist movement that is limited by adjustable friction. These wrists often only resist unwanted movement with light loads.
- Quick disconnect for externally powered TDs (without rotator)—This wrist provides a connection between a battery, control input(s) and an electric TD. Wrist rotation is possible through manual positioning of the TD (in other words, it has no battery powered wrist rotation). See Figure 15.20.

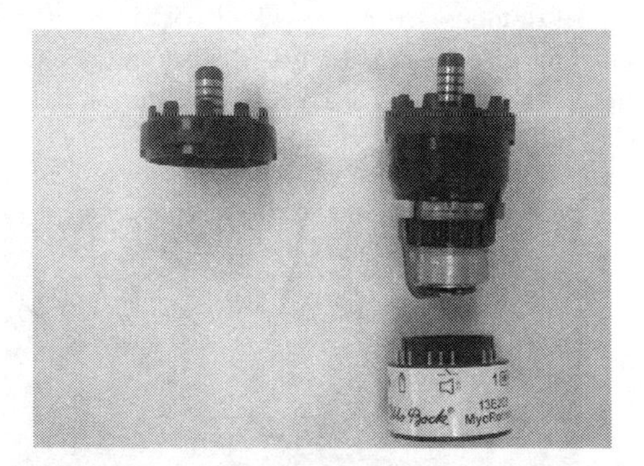

Figure 15.20 Quick disconnect wrist units for use with externally powered TDs. This picture shows the length difference between one with and without an electric wrist motor. The unit on the right has a motor for powered rotation. The component beneath it is a four-channel processor needed with this particular wrist rotator for certain TDs. In some cases, like that of externally powered WD prosthesis, the TD may be attached directly to the socket, without a wrist unit, to preserve length.

- Electric wrist rotator allows QD of the powered TD and provides the capability for powered wrist rotation. The motor and control for wrist rotation significantly adds length to the component, as seen in Figure 15.20. This is not used with WD cases and will usually not be used in the long TR cases either.

As shown in Figure 15.18–15.20, some wrist units come with multiple features or components that can be combined to gain more function. Unilateral WD cases, as mentioned earlier, offer a limited choice in regard to the selection of a wrist unit. In most scenarios, a QD style wrist unit, will not be advisable due to the length concerns discussed earlier in this chapter. In order to minimize the length of this component, in the case of an externally powered WD prosthesis, the TD may be directly attached to the socket frame without the use of a wrist unit. The TD can, however, still be rotated in space due to the ROM available with voluntary pronation/supination captured by the interface.

Terminal Devices

Terminal devices (TD) typically come in the form of either a hook or a hand, though there are some TDs that are commercially designed for special purposes, as seen in Figures 15.7 and 15.8. Other TDs can be custom-made for very specific purposes, if necessary.

Hooks are generally more durable and rugged than hands and allow finer prehension. Hands are more cosmetically appealing to most but they block the user's field of view while hooks have a more open design, allowing the amputee to see more of what they are doing when using the TD. An amputee should have the opportunity to try each in order to make the best decision for what is right for them. However, every amputee should receive multiple TDs, provided they show interest in doing so, as no single device can replace all of the lost functions that they once had with the anatomical hand.

There are hooks and hands designed for cable-driven as well as externally powered devices. Examples of each are shown in Figures 15.21 and 15.22. Terminal devices made for use with cable-driven prostheses are classified as either voluntary opening (VO) or voluntary closing (VC).

VO devices allow the user to open the TD when tension is applied to the control cable of the harness. As tension is increased on the control strap of the harness, the elastic bands or springs of the TD is overcome to allow the device to open. The potential energy within the elastic bands or springs will work to close the TD

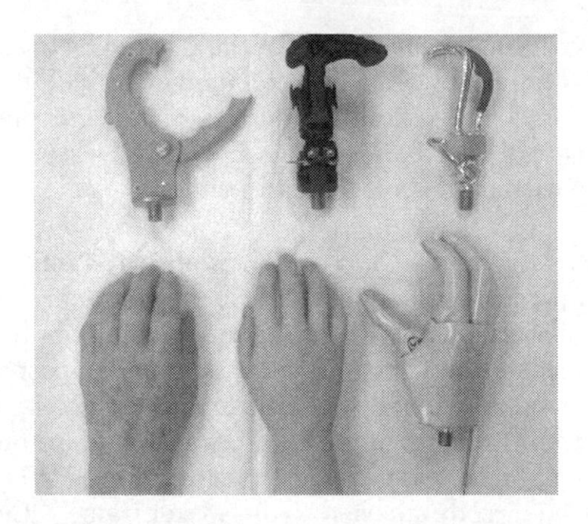

Figure 15.21 Sample of TDs that do not require battery power. Clockwise from top left: TRS Grip (VC), V2P hook (VO), 5XA hook (VO), APRL hand (VC), prefabricated semi-prehensile MCV-coated hand, and a custom silicone hand.

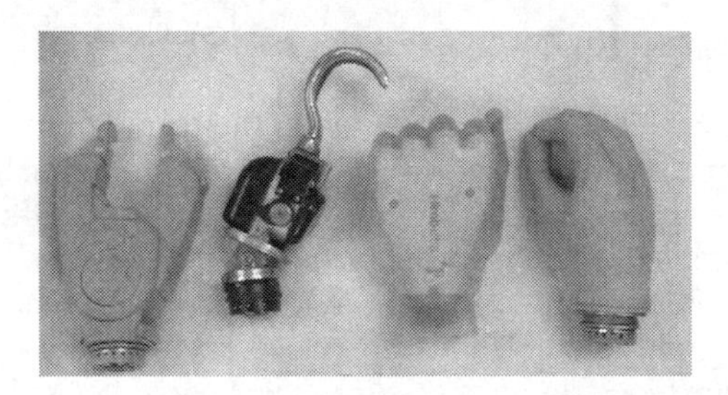

Figure 15.22 Sample of powered TDs. From left to right: Greifer, ETD with flexion unit, I-Limb Ultra multi-articulated hand, and the DMC plus.

as tension in the harness is relieved. The pinch force of this type of TD is not controlled by the user but rather by the tension stored in the elastic bands or springs. The advantage of this is that the amputee does not have to maintain tension on the harness while holding an object with the TD. Some hooks allow the user to change the pinch force, without adding elastic bands, by flipping a lever, as in the "Sierra 2 load" hook, or sliding a ratchet mechanism as in the V2P hook seen on the prosthesis shown in Figures 15.16, 15.19, and 15.21.

VC devices utilize the same body motions used to operate the VO TDs except that the motion results in closing the TD. These devices give the amputee more proportional control of the grip force. The more the tension applied through the harness, the stronger the grip. The disadvantage is that the tension needs to be applied continuously in order to maintain the same grip force. This can become tiresome and difficult for the user. There are, however, locking mechanisms, as in the case with the Army Prosthetics Research Laboratory (APRL) VC hand, and modifications to control cables that can be done, to allow the TD to be fixed in a given closed position but the force of the grip force may not be necessarily maintained.

Voluntary closing devices are more often considered in prostheses for amputations resulting in longer TR or WD limbs, than for those of shorter ones. This is due to the comparative increase in range of motion and strength remaining in the residual limb, which allows this population to better use this design. However, overall, VO TDs are still used more frequently than VC devices.

As previously mentioned, externally powered TDs also come in the form of hooks or hands. The traditional externally powered TDs allow the user to open and close the TD using a control input, usually a myoelectric signal picked up by an electrode embedded in the prosthetic interface. The speed and pinch force are proportionally controlled by the strength and duration of the control signal. Traditional devices do not offer the user the ability to utilize various grip patterns; the hooks simply open and close. Traditional versions of the externally powered hand open and close in a three-jaw chuck pattern. The only movement that occurs is that between the thumb and the index/ring finger. When compared to each other, externally powered hooks and hands have the same advantages and disadvantages in regard to the field of view, during functional activities, as do their cable-driven counterparts. However, in recent years, a new class of powered hands has emerged, the multi-articulated, powered hand. These hands allow movement in each finger, some even having individual motors for each digit. The thumb is also articulated to allow it to be oriented in a "non-opposed" position, which allows alternate grip patterns such as the lateral pinch grip. The multi-articulated hands have the advantage of being more anthropomorphic than the standard powered hand and allow the user to use various grip patterns.

There are WD versions of some of the externally powered hands, including some of the multi-articulated models. To minimize the added length, these designs are made to be directly mounted on the socket and do not allow the user to have the QD option. This would require a separate prosthesis for each powered TD, should more than one type be indicated.

SUMMARY

Wrist disarticulations and amputations resulting in long TR limbs, provide several advantages to the amputee: they preserve a significant amount of anatomical pronation/supination; provide more forearm leverage than that of shorter amputations, which preserves strength for elbow flexion; and allow for lower trimlines in the prosthetic interface, which increases the functional ROM with the prosthesis. The trimlines can be modified based on the intended use: for more rugged use, the ulna side trimline should terminate at or close to the olecranon; for lighter duty use, the trimlines can terminate at the distal third of the limb.

The disadvantages, relating to fitting of prostheses for the long TR or WD amputee, include the limited selection of functional components. Wrist units that provide features such as flexion, QD, and/or powered rotation may not be appropriate due to the resulting added length of the prosthesis.

It is ideal to allow the amputee to try out different interface designs and components during the trial fitting period before a definitive design is selected.

If the amputee's main goal is that of aesthetic appeal, then a self-suspending, semi-prehensile cosmetic prosthesis should be considered, including the option of a custom silicone hand.

If the amputee would like something that is cosmetically appealing with a broader range of function than that of the semi-prehensile design, then a myoelectric device may be considered. However, the added length resulting from the use of an electric wrist rotator disqualifies it from the consideration for this population. In order to improve the chances of a successful outcome for an externally powered prosthesis, the patient must have at least one viable muscle signal in the forearm, have access to a prosthetic facility experienced with these devices, be willing to commit to training, and have adequate funding sources as these devices are expensive and may require frequent maintenance. Externally powered hands may also receive custom silicone gloves for added cosmetic appeal.

If the prosthesis is intended for heavy duty use, then a body powered design with the following features should be considered.

- Harness: figure-of-eight or shoulder saddle harness, with flexible elbow hinges, to allow maximum ROM for pronation/supination.
- Interface: posterior interface trimlines that terminate at, or near, the olecranon for maximum dispersion of force load.

- Wrist unit: either a low profile wrist unit (for the long TRs), or none at all (for WDs).
- Terminal device: an appropriate hook or specialty TD.
- A forearm cuff, with or without a QD adapter, should be considered for all amputees at this level as they are inexpensive, lightweight, durable and easy to use. They provide a very good functional alternative to a full prosthesis when the individual does not feel like wearing a prosthesis.

Every prescription should be focused on addressing the patient's goals. Each patient needs to be educated on the options available, so that realistic expectations can be set and the appropriate course can be decided upon. A team, including an experienced prosthetist, should meet with the patient to address questions and concerns. Each patient should be willing to comply with the necessary training that may be involved with the prescription of a particular device before it is seriously considered. The prescription of multiple devices is encouraged for those who are active and experienced with the use of a prosthesis. As described earlier in this chapter, these secondary devices may be designed for a specific function or just be made as a spare device to provide a functional alternative, should the primary prosthesis need repair.

Clear communication between the patient, prosthetist, therapist, and physician, relating to all appropriate options, in regard to prostheses, will provide a basis for realistic expectations and enhance the chance of a successful outcome in improving the quality of life for the upper limb amputee.

REFERENCES

1. Raichle KA, Hanley MA, Molton I, et al. Prosthesis use in persons with lower and upper limb amputation. *JRRD*. 2008;45(7):961–972.
2. Dillingham TR, Pezzin LE, Mackenzie EJ. Limb amputation and limb deficiency: Epidemiology and recent trends in the United States. *South Med J*. 2002;95(8):875–883.
3. National Limb Loss Information Center. Amputation statistics by cause. Limb loss in the United States. NLLIC fact sheet. 2008. Available at: www.amputeecoalition.org/fact_sheets/amp_stats_cause.pdf. Accessed February 6, 2012.
4. Hartigan BJ, Sarrafian SK. Kinesiology and Functional Characteristics of the Upper Limb. In: Smith DG, Michael JW, Bowker JH, eds. *Atlas of Amputations and Limb Deficiencies – Surgical, Prosthetic and Rehabilitation Principles*, 3rd ed. American Academy of Orthopedic Surgeons; 2004, pp. 101–116.

5. Jones LE, Davidson JH. Save that arm: A study of problems in the remaining arm of unilateral upper limb amputees. *Prosthet Orthot Int.* 1999;23:55–58.
6. Reddy MP. Nerve entrapment syndromes in the upper extremity contralateral to amputation. *Arch Phys Med Rehabil.* 1984;65:24–26.
7. Wright TW, Hagan AD, Wood MB. Prosthetic usage in major upper extremity amputations. *J Hand Surgery [Am].* 1995;20(4):619–622.
8. Dudkiewicz I, Gabrielov R, Seiv-Ner I, et al. Evaluation of prosthetic usage in upper limb amputees. *Diabil Rehabil.* 2004;26(1):60–63.
9. Childress DS, Weir RF. Control of limb prostheses. In: Smith DG, Michael JW, Bowker JH, eds. *Atlas of Amputations and Limb Deficiencies – Surgical, Prosthetic and Rehabilitation Principles*, 3rd ed. American Academy of Orthopedic Surgeons; 2004:188.
10. Miguelez J, Conyers D, Macjulian L, Gulick K. Upper extremity prosthetics. In: Pasquina PF, Cooper RA, eds. *Textbooks of Military Medicine: Care of the Combat Amputee*. The Office of the Surgeon General at TMM Publications; 2009:614.
11. Fairly M. Osseointegration in the wave of the future. The O&P Edge. Sept, 2006. Available at: http://www.oandp.com/articles/2006-09_03.asp. Accessed May 21, 2012.
12. Hartigan BJ, Sarrafian SK. Kinesiology and functional characteristics of the upper limb. In: Smith DG, Michael JW, Bowker JH, eds. *Atlas of Amputations and Limb Deficiencies – Surgical, Prosthetic and Rehabilitation Principles*, 2nd ed. American Academy of Orthopedic Surgeons, 1992, reprinted 2002. Available at: http://www.oandplibrary.org/alp/chap05-01.asp. Accessed May 21, 2012.
13. Taylor CI. The biomechanics of control in upper extremity prosthetics. *Artificial Limbs.* 1955;2(3):14. Available at: http://www.oandplibrary.org/al/1955_03_004.asp. Accessed May 26, 2012.

RESOURCES

Meier RH, Atkins DJ. Functional Restoration of Adults and Children with Upper Extremity Amputation. *Demos Medical*, 2004.

Muzumdar A. Powered Upper Limb Prostheses—Control, Implementation and Clinical Application. *Springer-Verlag Berlin Heidelberg*, 2004.

Pasquina PF, Cooper RA. Textbooks of Military Medicine: Care of the Combat Amputee. *The Office of the Surgeon General at TMM Publications*, 2009.

Smith DG, Michael JW, Bowker JH. Atlas of Amputations and Limb Deficiencies—Surgical, Prosthetic and Rehabilitation Principles, 3rd ed. *American Academy of Orthopedic Surgeons*, 2004.

16

Prosthetic Prescriptions for Short Transradial Amputations

Christopher Fantini

General concepts and considerations applicable to the prosthetic management of individuals with upper limb amputation were introduced in the previous chapter and should be reviewed accordingly. This chapter expands on those concepts and applies them to the prosthetic management of transradial amputations that result in shorter limbs. The short transradial limb is defined, for the purposes of this chapter, as one where up to 50% of the original length of the radius and ulna remain after amputation (see Figure 16.1). Though these amputations result in functional challenges to the amputee, the expectation for a functional outcome is still relatively high to those of a higher level amputation.

The general considerations and six prosthetic options discussed in the previous chapter also apply to short transradial cases. To review, these options are as follows: no prosthesis; semi-prehensile cosmetic design; body powered (cable-driven) design; externally powered design; hybrid design; and the specialty/task specific design.

The primary differences between the shorter transradial level amputation and the long/wrist disarticulation level, when considering the design of a prosthesis, reside in the interface/socket design and the expanded choice of components. The rehabilitation team,

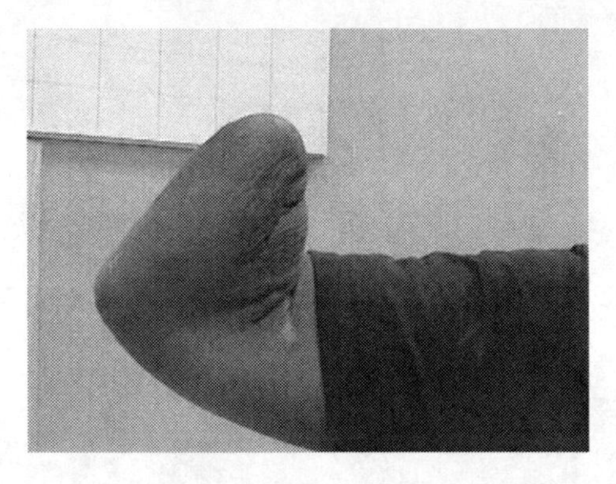

Figure 16.1 Picture of a short transradial residual limb in a flexed position.

including a prosthetist, should make the patient fully aware of the advantages and disadvantages of each choice considered so that the best interface design and combination of components are selected to fulfill the patient's goals.

PROSTHETIC CONSIDERATIONS

Muscle strength and range of motion (ROM) are adversely affected in shorter residual limbs. Elbow stability, active range of motion (AROM), specifically with elbow flexion, and weakness, due to loss of leverage, are all significant concerns to be addressed when considering a prosthetic design.

As a general rule, the shorter the residual limb, the more proximal the trimlines of the socket interface and frame need to be to maintain stability of the prosthesis with the limb. The term "trimline" refers to the proximal edges of the socket interface and frame. In body powered designs, rigid hinges, mounted on the outside of the socket frame, can be used to add stability. This allows the forces applied to the prosthesis to be distributed over a larger surface of the limb, reducing the load per unit area. This also improves contact, between the residuum and interface, for better suspension and improved medial/lateral stability at the elbow. There is no concern with the prosthesis limiting forearm pronation and supination since anatomical AROM is significantly reduced, or completely absent. As illustrated in Chapter 15, there are numerous prosthetic wrist components that will compensate for the motion lost.

Due to the short lever of the residual limb, care should be taken in keeping as much of the weight of the prosthesis as proximal to the elbow as possible. This will minimize the work required for the amputee to lift the prosthesis to flex the elbow. This can be done via the selection of lightweight components or by shortening the prostheses (as compared to what the normal limb length was prior to amputation). In addition to providing better leverage, shortening the prostheses also facilitates the ability of the user to perform activities at midline by making it easier to get the terminal device to the face or center of the body, where much of the activities of daily living (ADL) take place. Shortened prostheses are especially beneficial to the bilateral transradial amputee, as it improves their ability to perform ADL and makes them more independent.

External Power vs. Body Powered Designs

If the primary goal for the use of the prosthesis is to provide a more aesthetic appeal with light duty function, then either a semi-prehensile cosmetic, or externally powered prosthesis should be considered. The externally powered design will offer the user many functional advantages over the semi-prehensile cosmetic design including active control of the terminal device, for grasping and releasing objects, as well as the option for powered wrist rotation (see Figure 16.2).

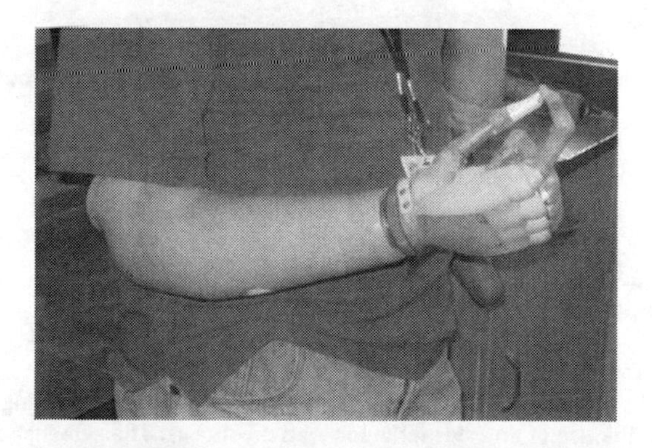

Figure 16.2 Example of a self-suspending, myoelectric prosthesis for a short, right, transradial limb. Interface is supracondylar in design. The terminal device is a first generation model I-Limb with a clear protective glove that also improves surface friction for grasping objects.

The externally powered device should only be given serious consideration if all of the prerequisites discussed in Chapter 15 are met. This includes a commitment on the part of the patient, to comply with the necessary training and trial fittings that are associated with externally powered prostheses. Testing and training for such devices include the use of myotesters (Figure 16.3) and software tools specific to the component that is being considered (examples shown in Figure 16.4).

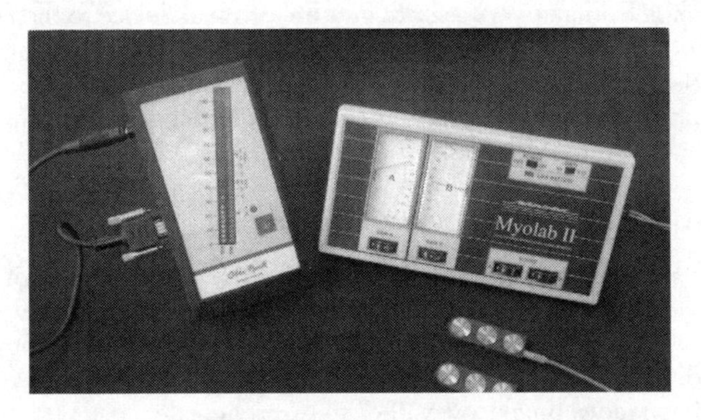

Figure 16.3 Examples of testing devices used to evaluate myoelectric signals. These devices can also be used to evaluate the signals from alternative control input devices such as linear transducers or force sensitive resistors.

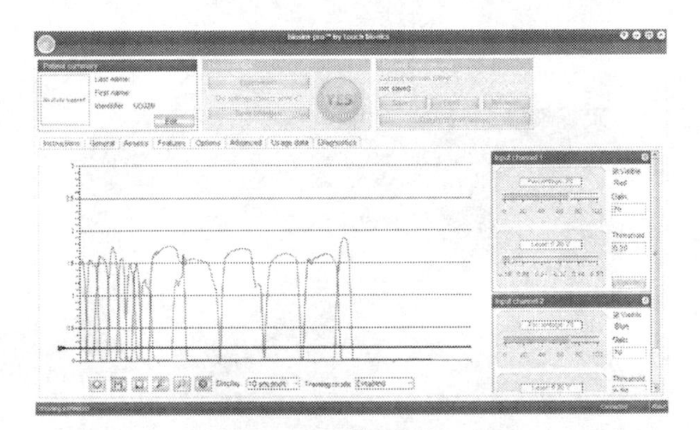

Figure 16.4 Example of the software used for setting up and training the amputee in the use of an externally powered prosthesis. The screenshot of the BioSim software package for the I-Limb Ultra prosthetic hand (by Touch Bionics), shows the strength and duration of the myoelectric signal generated by the amputee. The software can be used to test and train the potential candidate for an externally powered prosthesis.

When the amputee wishes to have a prosthesis that is designed for more rugged, heavy duty activities that cause significant torque about the elbow, a body powered, cable driven prosthesis, is the most appropriate choice since it offers the most effective design for improving/protecting stability at the elbow. In this case, the prosthesis should include rigid outside hinges, with harness suspension, to maximize comfort in absorbing the forces through the prosthesis and maximize stability about the elbow.

Elbow Hinges for Transradial Prostheses

Elbow hinges are divided into two categories, flexible and rigid. The hinges attach to either a triceps pad, a half cuff, or a full cuff around the humerus.

Flexible hinges are indicated for longer residual limbs and favored for body powered designs involving bilateral transradial amputees, as they allow the widest ROM, including that of any pronation/supination that may remain. Flexible hinges are the most common type of hinge used with transradial, body powered prostheses.

Rigid hinges are indicated in body powered prostheses for short residual limbs, as defined earlier, as well as prostheses intended for heavy duty use. They protect the very short residuum from excessive torque and prevent rotation of the socket on the limb, but do not allow any anatomical pronation/supination. Rigid hinges are traditionally avoided for bilateral transradial amputees (except in special cases as described below) or whenever anatomical pronation/supination needs to be preserved.

There are four basic types of rigid hinges for transradial level prostheses: single-axis hinges, polycentric hinges, step-up hinges, and limb-activated locking hinges. Each has unique features that make them favorable under various circumstances.

- Single-axis hinges are the simple design used for the short-to-mid-length limb. They are indicated for heavy duty use with limbs that have enough ROM and strength at the elbow to use the terminal device near the face and midline.
- Polycentric hinges are good for short residual limbs with muscle weakness which can limit elbow flexion. The center of rotation changes with the flexion angle making it relatively easier to flex the elbow.
- Step-up hinges are recommended for very short transradial amputations with redundant tissue, or bilaterals who lack sufficient ROM for elbow flexion to get the terminal device to the face. Every degree of flexion in the anatomical elbow will result in 2 or more

degrees of flexion at the hinge, allowing the user to improve their reach to midline or their face, with the terminal device. This extra ROM comes at the cost of the extra strength required to flex the elbow.

- Limb-activated locking hinges allow the user to lock the elbow in one of five positions of flexion. This is an option for the very short amputee who lacks the strength to carry loads or hold objects with a flexed elbow for extended durations of time.

Harness Designs

There are three basic harness designs used with body powered prostheses: the figure-of-nine harness (used with self-suspending prostheses), the figure-of-eight design (the most commonly used harness), and the shoulder saddle with chest strap (good for heavy duty use or those who cannot take the pressure in the sound side axilla region, exerted by either the figure-of-eight or figure-of-nine harness). Further discussion on harness design can be found in Chapter 15 otherwise refer to [1] for detailed information on various harness styles.

Self-Suspending Interfaces

Typically, self-suspended interface designs for the short transradial amputee are used for light duty prostheses such as the semi-prehensile cosmetic design or an externally powered design. As was described in Chapter 15, the self-suspending interface can be held onto the transradial residual limb by either using contours designed over the humeral epicondyles (supracondylar suspension) or by creating a suction environment between the limb and interface (via an intimate fit with a one-way air expulsion valve incorporated into the interface, or using silicone/gel roll-on liners or sleeves).

Supracondylar Suspension

Supracondylar suspension will result in some loss of ROM at the elbow since the interface crosses the elbow joint. However, the loss can be mitigated by using flexible materials and or window cut-outs over the frame and epicondyles (see Figure 16.5). In addition, the alignment of the wrist can be pre-flexed on the forearm during fabrication, to orient the terminal device toward midline. Components that allow motion for locking wrist flexion and/or rotation may also be used to accommodate minor loss in elbow ROM and improve the ability of the amputee to get the terminal device to midline and the face.

There are a number of variations to supracondylar, self-suspending, designs for the short transradial residual limb. Generally, they all favor a *pull-in* donning method where the amputees pull their limb into the socket interface, using a pull sheath or stocking, in order to ensure maximum contact between the interface and limb. The shorter the limb, the more important it is to get as much tissue as possible into the interface to maximize comfort, stability, and control. This is in contrast to the donning method employed with designs for the longer residual limbs, which include the amputee *pushing* their limb into the socket. Modifications can be made, particularly for the case of the short transradial bilateral amputee, to allow them to use the *push-in* method to don the interface, as this is easier to accomplish for the bilateral amputee. However the push-in technique usually results in less stability between the prosthesis and limb than with the *pull-in* method of donning. The three styles discussed below are described in literature and can be considered for the short transradial limb. Other variations may be used by individual practitioners.

The Muenster interface is a classic design and described in multiple texts while the Anatomically Contoured and Controlled Interface (ACCI) and the Compression/Release Stabilized interface (CRS) represent more recent designs [2–5]. A summary of their general features follows:

- The Muenster style socket: used for very short, fleshy limbs; indicated for light duty prostheses, like the semi-prehensile cosmetic or externally powered designs; characterized by anterior/posterior pressure in the cubital fold and distal triceps tendon (just above the olecranon).
- The ACCI combines features of Northwestern and Muenster styles to try to improve comfort, stability and suspension. It is also characterized by anterior/posterior pressure but with additional channels of pressure along the anterior aspect of the radius and posterior aspect of the ulna. There is also pressure applied to the medial and lateral aspect of the biceps tendon. A very similar socket design is described in the literature as the Transradial Anatomically Contoured Interface (TRAC) [2,3].
- The CRS interface (also referred to as the High-Fidelity Interface) attempts to maximize skeletal stabilization within the socket in order to allow more efficiency and greater ROM. This is accomplished by alternating areas of high tissue compression with areas of tissue release. The tissue is released through either window cut-outs of the socket, as shown in Figure 16.5, or with reliefs built into the thermoflexible interface [4,5].

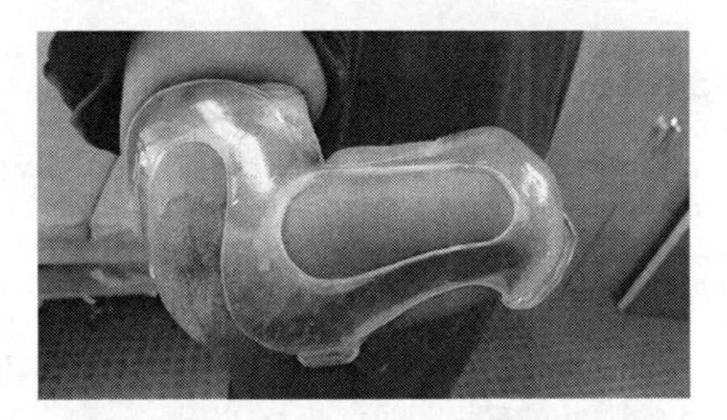

Figure 16.5 A clear, thermoplastic test socket showing the CRS interface with windowed cut-outs. Test sockets, aka diagnostic sockets, are usually made of a low cost, clear, semi-rigid or rigid thermoplastic material and allow the patient and prosthetist to assess the fit and comfort of the socket interface prior to fabricating the final product. The definitive interface is made once a satisfactory result is achieved with the test fitting.

Suction/Liner Suspension

Roll-on liners or sleeves can provide an effective suspension method for the unilateral, short transradial amputee (see example in Figure 16.6). However, compromised function in the sound hand/limb, may disqualify the use of a roll-on liner or sleeve if it results in too much difficulty with donning for the amputee. Caution is advised in using liners and sleeves in bilateral cases, due to the obvious difficulty with donning that would result for this population as well.

Suspension via suction with a one-way air expulsion valve, incorporated into the thermoflexible interface, may be used but should be augmented with a suspension sleeve as suction on its own, with a very short limb is usually inadequate.

The disadvantages of using roll-on liners or sleeves are the added bulk, weight, and heat retention that result. In addition these items need to be cleaned daily and replaced every 3 to 6 months, depending on wear, adding additional recurring expense.

Wrist Units

All available wrist options, including those described in Chapter 15, can be considered for a prosthesis made for the short transradial amputee. In unilateral cases, where more than one terminal device may be used, the quick disconnect locking wrist unit is a good option. This device also locks the position of the terminal device (TD) to prevent any unwanted rotation during active use.

Individuals with functional deficits on the sound side, as well as those with bilateral upper limb amputations, may also benefit from

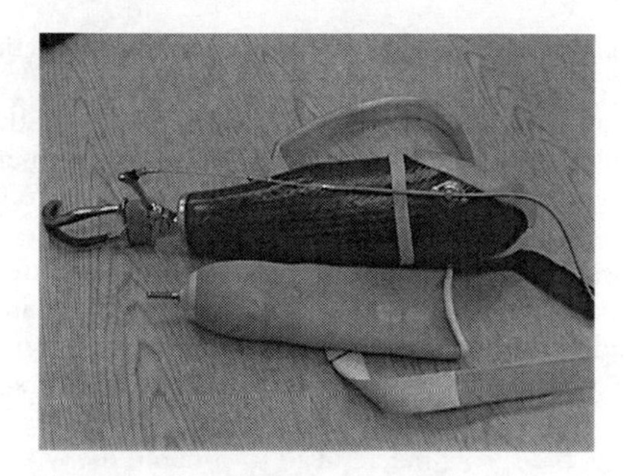

Figure 16.6 Photo shows a body powered transradial prosthesis. A silicone locking liner sits adjacent to the prosthesis.

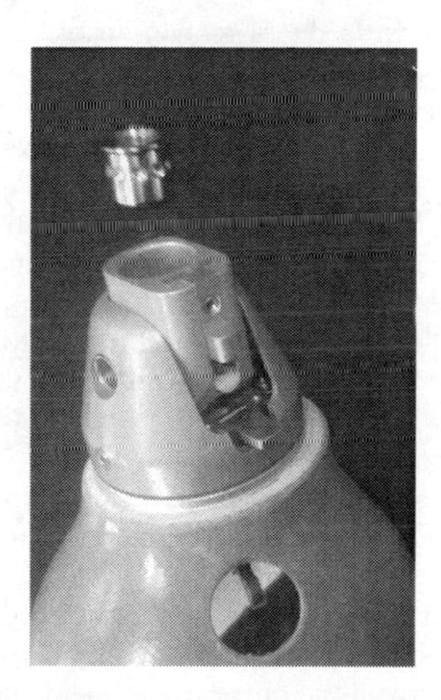

Figure 16.7 The Texas Assistive Devices Five Function Wrist. This wrist features quick disconnection of the terminal device with locking rotation at the connection point, as well as a separate rotation axis at the base of the wrist unit. It is the proximal axis that is spring loaded to pronate upon release of the lock, which is seen in the circular cut-out of the interface frame. This unit also allows wrist flexion.

the use of a wrist flexion feature, to increase their functional range of activity.

Some non-powered wrist units, like the Texas Assistive Devices model in Figure 16.7, come with spring mechanisms that allow the user to actively control wrist rotation. This is can be done with the control cable on the terminal device by releasing the wrist rotation lock, using either a paddle switch, separate control cable, or the contralateral limb. While the lock is released, the amputee can freely control wrist rotation by countering the spring force (which is directed toward pronation) with tension on the cable attached to the TD. Increasing tension will supinate the wrist while easing cable tension will allow the spring mechanism to pronate the wrist. Once the desired rotation is achieved, the wrist can be easily locked in position by allowing the rotation lock to re-engage.

When externally powered devices are used, it is beneficial to incorporate a powered wrist rotator to allow the amputee to regain pronation/supination capabilities. Rotation is usually operated via myoelectric control with the forearm flexors set to pronate and extensors set to supinate the wrist. A method of switching myoelectric control to/from the hand and wrist may include co-contraction of the antagonistic muscle pair or the control could be dictated by speed and intensity of contraction where a less intense contraction would be assigned control in the operation of the terminal device and a forceful contraction would control wrist function. For example, mild contraction of the forearm flexors could be used to close the hand while a more forceful contraction be used to pronate the wrist. This requires a lot of skill on the part of the amputee. A third option for switching control from the wrist to the hand would be the use of an external switch.

Optional features, such as passive wrist flexion/extension and radial/ulnar deviation, are also compatible with externally powered wrist rotators; however, these added features currently come attached to a select group of externally powered terminal devices, as is seen in the electric terminal device (ETD) in Figure 16.8, and are not inherent in any of the currently available powered wrist units themselves. Powered wrist flexion/extension units are being developed, but are not yet commercially available; as of the time of this writing.

In addition to flexion and extension, passive radial and ulnar deviation options, such as with the MultiFlex Wrist Unit from Motion Control Inc, are also available for both powered and non-powered devices.

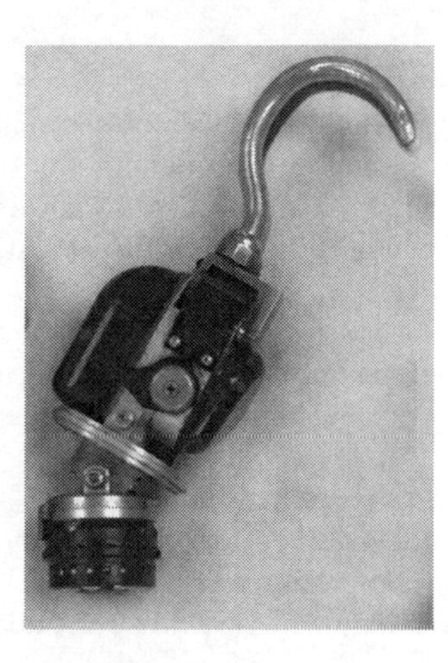

Figure 16.8 The ETD with optional wrist flexion feature, by Motion Control Inc. The terminal device can be positioned and locked in various positions of flexion and extension.

Transradial Hybrid Design—Wrist Adapter to Allow Use of Body Powered TDs With Electric Wrist

There may be cases when an individual would like to switch from an externally powered TD to a body powered one without having to switch prostheses or other cases where the individual prefers the function of an externally powered wrist rotator with a cable operated terminal device. A wrist adapter is available that allows an externally powered prosthesis to be converted into a hybrid without having to doff the prosthesis. Powered wrist rotation is maintained, but the adapter allows any terminal device, with a threaded stud connector, to connect to the rotator (see Figure 16.9).

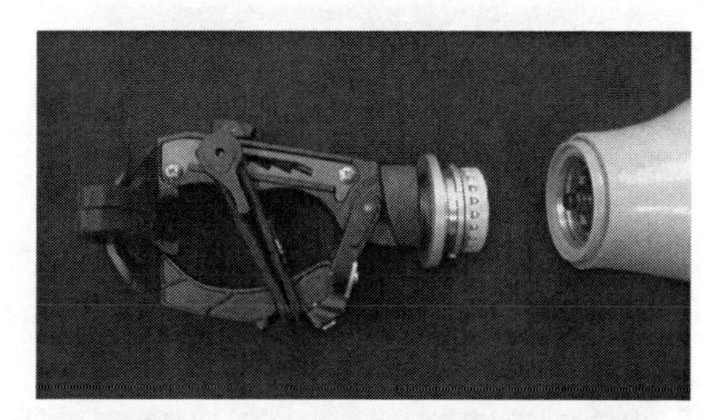

Figure 16.9 Wrist adapter which allows body powered terminal devices, like the V2P hook, to be connected to an externally powered wrist.

Terminal Devices

Body powered designs for the short transradial population often incorporate the use of voluntary opening (VO) terminal devices. Short residual limbs make it more difficult to efficiently use voluntary closing devices, which require more ROM, strength, and muscle stamina than VO devices.

In bilateral cases, hooks can provide more functional value as they are lighter, allow for finer prehension, and maximize the user's field of view when grasping and releasing objects as compared to prosthetic hands.

Externally powered terminal devices have advanced in recent years and now include choices for multi-articulated or dexterous hands. These include components such as the I-Limb Ultra (by Touch Bionics), the BeBionic hand (by RSLSteeper), and the Michelangelo hand (by Otto Bock).

Externally powered multi-articulated hands offer more variety in grip patterns than the traditional electric hands. Multi-articulated hands differ from their predecessors in two significant ways – all of the fingers in the externally powered multi-articulated hand actively flex/extend and they possess two axes of movement in the thumb.

Traditional electric hands only allow powered movement at one joint, that between the thumb and the index/middle finger assembly (which is linked together to function as one unit). The ring and pinky finger are just foam fillers that do not actively move. In addition, the thumb is not designed to move out of the opposed position. The result is a single grip in a simple three-jaw chuck pattern (see Figure 16.10).

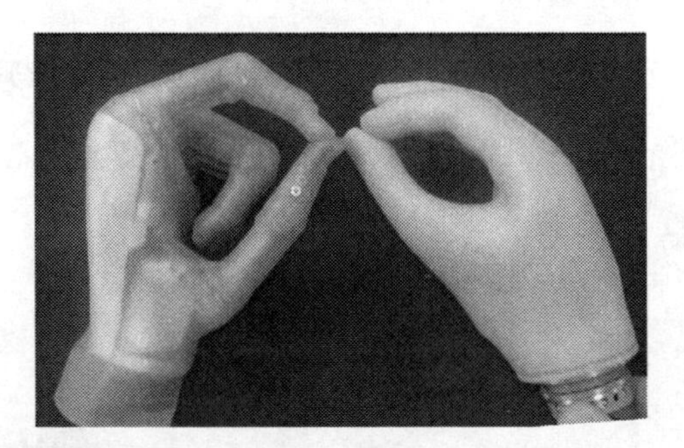

Figure 16.10 Multi-articulated hand (I-Limb Ultra) on left and traditional powered hand (Otto Bock DMC) on the right. Comparison of finger position in a fully closed position.

On the other "hand," the multi-articulated designs allow the use of multiple finger patterns such as lateral pinch, various versions of fine pinch, or a finger point orientation, which can be used to push buttons on a keyboard or phone (Figure 16.11). The software package, called BioSim, affiliated with the I-Limb Ultra hand, even allows the prosthetist to create a customized grip pattern in addition to selecting patterns that have been pre-programmed by the manufacturer (Figure 16.12).

See Chapter 15 for more discussion on terminal devices.

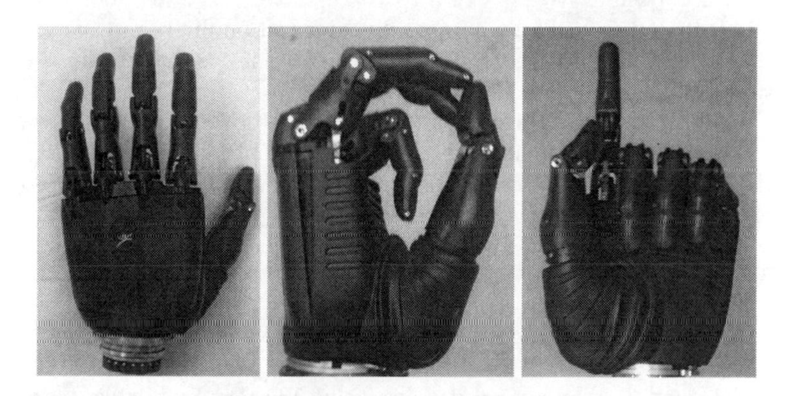

Figure 16.11 BeBionic hand examples of different grip patterns possible. From left to right—"relaxed" position, "three-jaw chuck" pattern, and "finger point" pattern. All fingers are capable of powered movement and the thumb can be manually positioned in an "opposed" or "unopposed" orientation, to increase the number of grip options.

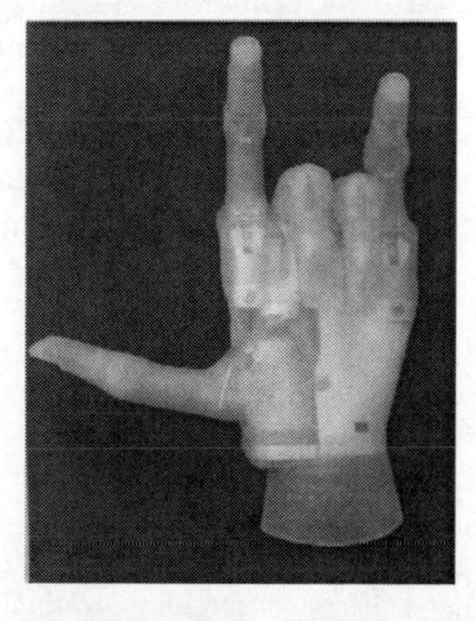

Figure 16.12 I-Limb Ultra in a custom programmed finger orientation.

SUMMARY

Prosthetic interface designs for the short transradial residual limb must address medial/lateral and rotary stability about the elbow and limb. This can be done using rigid outside hinges, with a harness suspended body powered design, for prostheses intended for heavy duty use. Lighter duty prostheses, such as semi-prehensile and externally powered designs can be suspended on the limb using contoured interface designs which extend over epicondyles and olecranon, eliminating the need for a harness. Locking roll-on liners and suction sleeves may also be used either on their own, or combined with the supracondylar interface designs.

Short transradial amputations result in the elimination of all anatomical wrist and hand functions including pronation/supination. However, a wide variety of prosthetic components are available to allow the amputee to regain wrist motion.

Hybrid design is available at the transradial level, though not used often, via a wrist adapter that will allow body powered TD to operate with an externally powered wrist rotator. Powered wrist flexion units are not yet commercially available but are being developed.

Though body powered devices, using VO terminal devices, are probably still the most widely used prosthetic option, the recent emergence of externally powered, multi-articulating hands have increased interest in myoelectric devices. These hands have more anthropomorphic movement than their predecessors and have increased the functional envelope of the prosthesis by enabling the use of various grasp patterns. Some devices have software packages that even allow the prosthetist to program a customized pattern for the patient.

Technology is advancing at a rapid pace. It is incumbent on members of the rehabilitation team to stay educated on the current state of the science so that the best service can be offered to the patient in need.

REFERENCES

1. Pursley RJ. Harness patterns for upper-extremity prostheses. *Artificial Limbs*. 1955;2(3):26–60. Available at: http://www.oandplibrary.org/al/1955_03_026.asp. Accessed May 29, 2012.
2. Alley RD. Advancement of upper extremity prosthetic interface and frame design. In: *Proceedings of UNB Myoelectric Controls/Powered Prosthetic*

Symposium, 2002; Fredericton, Canada: University of New Brunswick; 2002, pp. 28–32.

3. Miguelez JM, Lake C, Conyers D, Zenie J. The transradial anatomically contoured interface: Design principles and methodology. *J Prosthet Orthot*. 2003;15(4):148–156. Available at http://www.oandp.org/jpo/library/2003_04_148.asp
4. Alley RD, Williams TW, Albuquerque MJ, Altobelli DE. Prosthetic sockets stabilized by alternating areas of tissue compression and release. *J Rehabil Res Dev*. 2011;48(6):676–679.
5. http://www.biodesigns.com. Accessed May 29, 2012.

ADDITIONAL INFORMATION

- Website with general information about orthotics and prosthetics: http://www.oandp.com
- American Academy of Orthotists and Prosthetists: http://www.oandp.org/
- Otto Bock – (manufacturer of upper extremity prosthetic components including the Michelangelo hand): http://ottobockus.com/cps/rde/xchg/ob_us_en/hs.xsl/4713.html
- Motion Control – (manufacturer of externally powered prosthetic components): http://www.utaharm.com/index.php
- Liberating Technologies – (manufacturer of upper extremity prosthetic components): http://liberatingtechnologies.com
- TRS – (manufacturer of body powered and specialty prosthetic components): http://www.oandp.com/products/trs
- Texas Assistive Devices – (manufacturer of upper limb prosthetic components): http://n-abler.org
- Touch Bionics – (manufacturer of the I-Limb hand): http://www.touchbionics.com
- RSLSteeper – (manufacturer of upper extremity prosthetic components including the Bebionic hand): http://bebionic.com
- http://dukespace.lib.duke.edu/dspace/bitstream/handle/10161/4752/68%20Schulz.pdf?sequence=1 – (First Experiences with the Vincent Hand).
- http://upperlimbprosthetics.info
- http://arm-amp.com

17

Prosthetic Prescriptions for Transhumeral Amputations

Christopher Fantini

Many of the common principles in prosthetics management for any upper extremity amputation level have been covered in Chapters 15 and 16. Brief descriptions of surgical procedures, fitting concepts and prosthetic designs, specific to the transhumeral level of amputation, are discussed in this chapter, to better inform the reader of prosthetic prescription rationale. However, detailed discussion of these topics lies beyond the scope of this text. The reader should refer to the publications cited in the references, as well as the additional resources and websites, located at the end of the chapter, for further information.

INTRODUCTION

As with any amputation, there are multiple factors that determine successful outcomes in the prosthetic management of the transhumeral amputee. These include, but are not limited to, the type of surgery performed, residual limb length, pain, skin condition of the residual limb, strength in the limb, range of motion (ROM) remaining in the upper body, patient's motivation, patient's access to a multidisciplinary rehabilitation team including that of an experienced prosthetist, and the source of funding. Limb length, presence of pain, ROM, and strength in the residuum all have a direct impact on the patient's function with a prosthesis.

SURGICAL TECHNIQUES

In addition to the myoplasty, myodesis, cineplasty and osseointegration techniques briefly described in Chapter 15, surgical options for transhumeral level amputations include the following.

Angulation Osteotomy

The distal humerus is angulated to provide better suspension and rotational control of the prosthesis (see Figure 17.1). This technique can be used with mid-length to long residual limbs and has been suggested for bilateral transhumeral amputees to facilitate voluntary humeral rotation and increase independence [1].

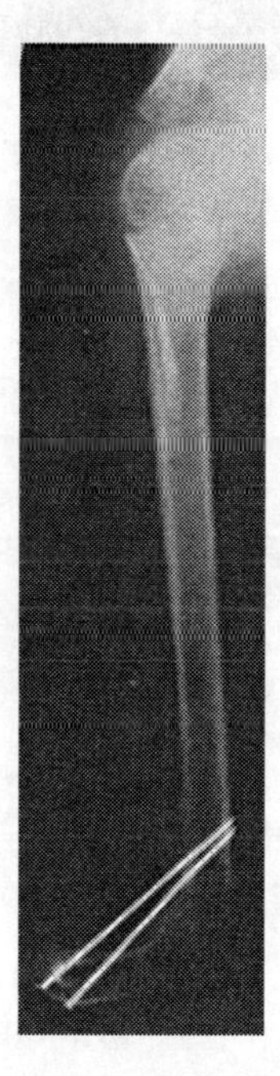

Figure 17.1 X-ray showing angulation osteotomy with a long transhumeral residuum.

Targeted Muscle Reinnervation (TMR)

Residual nerves from the amputated limb are transferred to muscle groups that no longer serve any mechanical function due to the amputation. The targeted muscle groups are denervated before the transfer

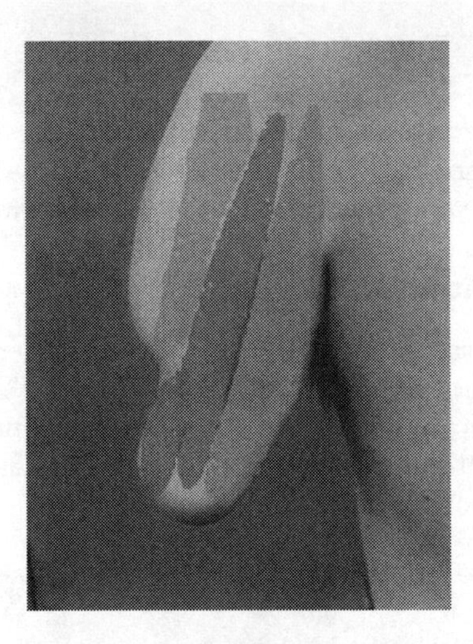

Figure 17.2 Photo highlighting the reinnervation strategy of transhumeral TMR surgery.

is performed and can be segmented to increase the potential number of new, individual muscle units. This surgery is currently performed for amputations done at the transhumeral, shoulder disarticulation, and scapulothoracic levels. As seen in the photo in Figure 17.2, transhumeral level TMR surgery includes transfer of the median nerve to the medial biceps (represented by the shaded highlight furthest right on the arm), the musculocutaneous nerve to the lateral biceps (represented by the shaded highlight in the center), the proximal radial nerve to the triceps (represented by the top, left shaded highlight), and the distal radial nerve to the brachialis (represented by the bottom left shaded highlight).

After a period of time, up to several months, the motor and sensory nerves reinnervate to the point where clear, independent, voluntary, muscle contractions are seen. The new voluntary muscle control can be used to operate four independent functions, in an externally powered prosthesis. These functions include flexing the elbow of a prosthesis with the lateral biceps, extending the elbow with the triceps, opening the hand with the brachialis (radial nerve), and closing the hand with the medial biceps (median nerve). Not only is the number of independently controlled myosites increased, it allows more intuitive control of the prosthesis as the amputee can use the same neural pathways that would have extended to the missing limb for similar functions. In other words, the patient has the potential to use the same thought patterns to operate the prosthesis that they would have for their own anatomical limb prior to the amputation.

In addition, the dermatome has been shown to change on the limb as the peripheral nerves reinnervate skin tissue as well. For example, pressure stimulus applied to an area on the skin above the biceps may be cognitively perceived by the amputee as pressure felt on their missing hand. Temperature stimulation shows similar results. In the future, these new sensory reinnervations may be utilized to provide sensory stimulus, for pressure and/or temperature, with prosthetic use [2–4].

Transhumeral amputations do result in enough space to use elbow units in a prosthesis. If the amputation results in a very short residual limb, such as one through the neck of humerus, then the amputee should be treated prosthetically, as a shoulder disarticulation case.

PROSTHETIC OPTIONS

The purpose of the prosthesis is to restore as much function as possible by expanding the amputee's "functional envelope" (see Chapter 15). This becomes increasingly difficult the higher the amputation level.

To review, the six prosthetics options for consideration of the upper extremity amputee are as follows (added features listed in parenthesis represent those specific for amputations above the elbow joint).

1. No prosthesis use.
2. Semi-prehensile cosmetic design (with a passive, lightweight endoskeletal elbow).
3. Body powered design (includes an elbow unit or outside locking hinges with a dual control harness). Example shown in Figure 17.3.
4. Externally powered design (includes a motorized elbow to allow powered flexion/extension). Example shown in Figure 17.6.
5. Hybrid design (includes use of a hybrid elbow unit which requires body power for flexion extension, has an electric locking mechanism, and is compatible with powered wrists/terminal devices).
6. Specialty/task specific designs (these may or may not include an actual elbow joint as they are made for specific activities).

All six options are appropriate for consideration in the case of the transhumeral amputee. However, only five options can be considered for the elbow disarticulated amputee, as externally powered elbow units are not practical with these cases.

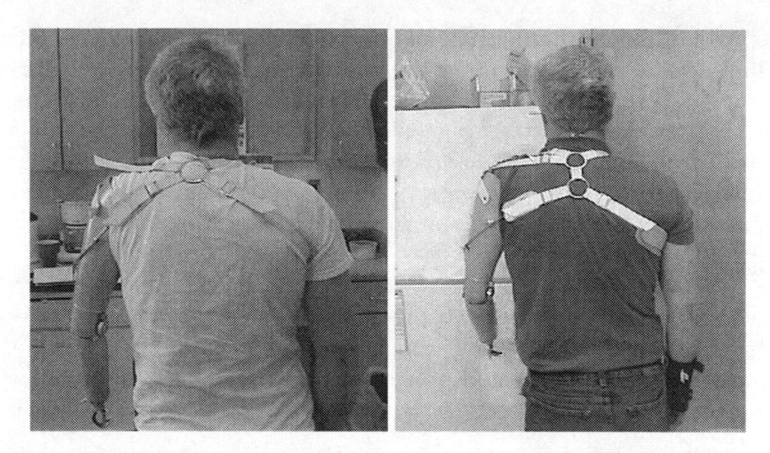

Figure 17.3 Figure-of-eight harness for a transhumeral body powered prosthesis. The harness on the left uses a single ring to transmit force through the harness on the back. If the ring slides up toward the neck during use, it reduces the amount of excursion in the control cable and can compromise function. It will also lead to discomfort. The harness on the right shows a double ring strategy which improves comfort and excursion by keeping the harness from riding up toward the neck.

In general, the same advantages and disadvantages for each of the six prosthetic options discussed in earlier chapters apply to the transhumeral and elbow disarticulation cases. Careful consideration and time should be devoted by the rehabilitation team to help the patient determine which design(s) is/are most appropriate for their specific case.

As with any upper extremity amputation, the fitting process and component selection for prosthetic devices at this level can take considerable time, effort, and expense. The patient must show strong interest and motivation for the process to be worthwhile. Testing different interface and component options during the early fitting phases of management will lead to better decisions in component and design selection, improving functional outcomes for the patient. In cases where the amputee becomes an active user or participates in activities that require a specific, separate design, then the prescription of multiple prostheses should be considered. Under most circumstances, active prosthetic users should have at least one spare prosthesis to maintain function, in case repairs are needed to the primary prosthesis. Spare prostheses are a necessity for the bilateral patient.

Prosthetic Consideration Based on Limb Length

A common theme among all amputation surgeries is the preservation of the maximum allowable length of the amputated limb. The idea is that the increased length will leave the amputee with as much natural function as possible in the residual limb and provide the maximum surface area and leverage possible to suspend and use a prosthesis, should one be used. The length of the limb will directly affect the type of prosthetic elbow considered for a prosthesis at the humeral level.

Elbow Disarticulation

Elbow disarticulations provide advantages for suspension and active humeral rotation of the prosthesis due to the preservation of the humeral epicondyles. This is particularly beneficial for bilateral amputees, for the same reason mentioned with angulation osteotomy, as the ability to actively control humeral rotation results in greater independence by expanding their functional envelope. Options, however, for prosthetic design are limited. Due to the length of the limb, there is not enough room to use either a normal or externally powered, prosthetic elbow unit. Outside locking elbow hinges are required for use with a prosthesis made for this level of amputation.

Outside locking hinges add weight as well as bulk to the prosthesis. The extra width resulting from the external hinges can limit clothing options for the wearer as tight fitting sleeves may not fit over the device.

Operation of the elbow is achieved through a dual control harness system. The term "dual control" refers to the two control cables controlled with the harness: (a) the elbow lock control cable, via the anterior elbow lock control strap; (b) the posterior control cable which either functions to enable flexion/extension of the elbow (when the elbow is unlocked) or operation of the TD (when the elbow is locked).

The body motions required for operating a dual control harness are as follows:

1. Elbow lock control—simultaneous humeral abduction, extension, and depression.
2. Elbow flexion—glenohumeral flexion, abduction, and biscapular abduction. The elbow must be unlocked to control elbow flexion/extension.
3. Operation of the TD—same motions as that for elbow flexion control; however the elbow must be locked to control the TD.

As of the time of this writing, externally powered elbows aren't used with elbow disarticulations, so the only battery powered design that may be considered is the hybrid, for this level of amputation. The elbow would be controlled as described above; however the wrist and/or terminal device can be operated with myoelectric control. The amputee can use various strategies to switch between wrist and hand control. Examples of switching strategies include, but are not limited to, co-contraction of antagonistic limb musculature or use of a toggle switch. Terminal devices are selected according to the assessment of the patient's desired use of the prosthesis.

Transhumeral Level

Transhumeral interface designs are usually harness-suspended but they can be self-suspended with the use of suction or with a roll-on liner system as described in Chapters 15 and 16. The compression/release stabilizing (CRS) interface design may also be considered (Figure 17.4). The harness-system can be that of the transhumeral figure-of-eight design (Figure 17.5), or a shoulder saddle and chest strap; both include an anterior control strap to operate the elbow lock, as seen in Figure 17.4.

Prosthetic elbow units are used for transhumeral level amputations. All transhumeral prosthetic elbow units (excluding outside

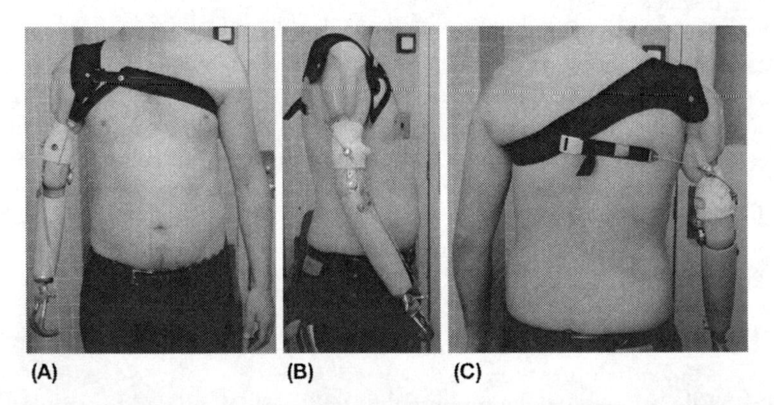

(A) (B) (C)

Figure 17.4 Picture shows (A) anterior, (B) lateral and (C) posterior view of a trial fitting of a transhumeral prosthesis featuring a shoulder saddle and chest strap harness, a test socket for a CRS interface, temporarily mounted to a body powered elbow (Positive Locking elbow by Hosmer) with an attached spring assist unit (on the medial axis of the elbow), and a voluntary opening hook.

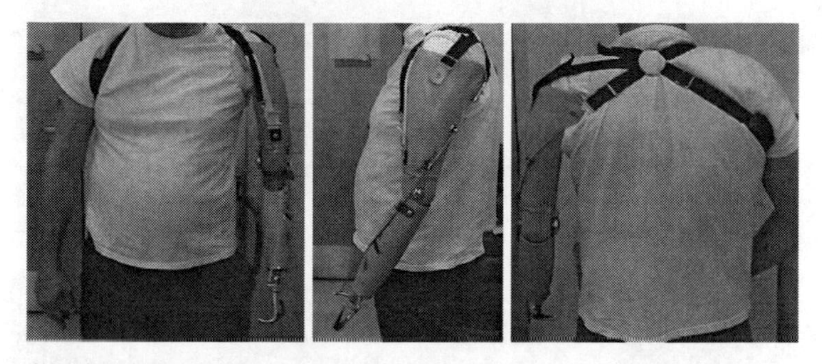

Figure 17.5 A definitive transhumeral body powered prosthesis with a dual control figure-of-eight harness, positive locking elbow with spring assist attachment, and voluntary opening hook.

locking hinges) allow two degrees of freedom: flexion/extension and humeral rotation.

1. Flexion/extension—controlled using one of the following methods: passive, manual manipulation, active control through a harness, or externally powered control via myoelectric, or switch control.
2. Humeral rotation—controlled by passive friction. Devices that provide an option of powered humeral rotation have been developed for clinical trials but are still not commercially available at the time of this writing [5].
3. Elbow units can be broken down into three categories: body powered, hybrid, and externally powered.
   a. Body powered designs require adequate strength and ROM in the residual limb to achieve the force and cable excursion necessary to operate the prosthesis. Examples include the Positive Locking Elbow (by Hosmer) and the Ergo Arm (by Otto Bock).

      The dual control harness, required to operate the body powered transhumeral prosthesis, functions as described earlier in the discussion of outside locking joints. If needed, additional components, such as an elbow flexion spring assist or forearm balance mechanism, may be used to reduce the force needed to flex the elbow.

      If the amputee has sufficient strength but lacks the excursion necessary to fully flex the elbow and/or operate the terminal device, an excursion amplifier may be added to the harness. Excursion amplifiers are small pulleys that double the amount of control cable excursion an amputee can gain from their normal ROM. This comes at the cost of the increased force required to operate the control cable. Typically, the shorter the limb, the less the excursion that is available. When the force and/or excursion available is not adequate enough to fully operate a body powered prosthesis efficiently, then either a hybrid or externally powered design is necessary.

b. Hybrid systems typically feature elbow units that use body power to control flexion/extension, with an electric elbow lock. Examples include the Utah Hybrid (by Motion Control) and the Ergo Hybrid (by Otto Bock). The terminal device and wrist are controlled via external power. This system provides a greater functional envelope than the body powered design but costs more, is heavier, and is not as durable. When compared to the externally powered design, it is less expensive, lighter, and provides faster elbow response; however sufficient ROM and strength are required to flex the elbow.

c. Externally powered elbow designs allow the option for sequential control of the powered motion of each joint or simultaneous powered control of the elbow and either the wrist or hand. Example shown in Figure 17.6.

Sequential control uses the same electric input signal to control the powered functions of the elbow, wrist and hand. A switching mechanism is employed to allow the user to cycle through the modes of control. For example, the same two electrode signals may be used, independently of each other, to control flexion/extension when the device is in elbow mode; pronation/supination when in wrist mode and open/close when in hand mode. The user can sequentially switch modes by using muscle co-contractions or an external switch.

Simultaneous control of the elbow and either the wrist or hand is ensured. Typically the elbow is controlled with either a linear transducer or strain gauge, attached to the harness and activated with the same motions used to control body powered elbows, glenohumeral flexion, abduction and/or biscapular abduction. The difference is that there is very little force or excursion necessary to activate the motor for elbow flexion. The elbow automatically locks once motion is stopped for a given period of time, which is adjustable in the

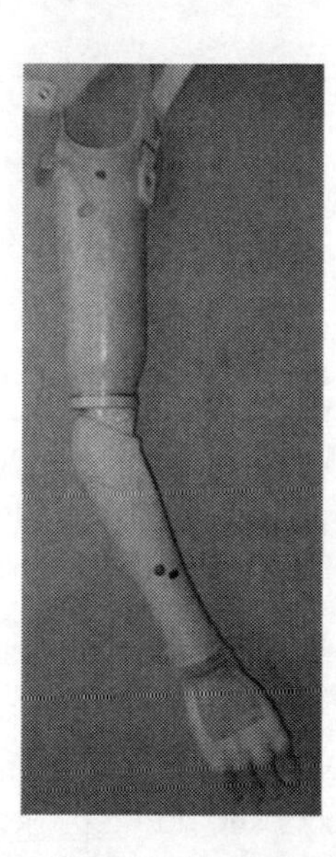

Figure 17.6 Externally powered transhumeral prosthesis featuring suction interface design, shoulder saddle and chest strap harness, electric elbow (Utah Arm by Motion Control), electric wrist rotator, and multi-articulating powered hand (I-Limb by Touch Bionics). A linear transducer, used to control powered elbow function, can be seen at the top left of the interface frame The amputee uses biscapular abduction or humeral flexion to apply tension to the transducer to activate control of the elbow.

software. The elbow unlocks automatically when tension is applied to the control input a second time. The wrist rotator and TD are typically controlled with dual site myoelectric inputs contained in the interface and placed over the biceps and triceps respectively. The same sequential control strategy mentioned above is used to allow the user to switch between wrist and hand mode.

Wrist Units and Terminal Devices

Example of prosthetic wrist units and terminal devices can be viewed in Chapters 15 and 16. The same components are available for use with the transhumeral level amputee. Any voluntary opening terminal device may be considered, both for the body powered and or hybrid designs. Voluntary closing terminal devices are contraindicated, for transhumeral and elbow disarticulation prosthetic devices, as there is insufficient ROM available to achieve the required cable excursion to fully operate the elbow and terminal device.

CONCLUSIONS

The prosthetic management of the transhumeral amputee is challenging. Establishing realistic expectations and goals is important in achieving success. In addition, consideration must be given to the needs and expectations of the patient's spouse, children or family. Once the goals and requirements are understood, an appropriate plan of rehabilitation can be formulated. This plan should include the opportunity for the amputee to test different devices and designs to determine what works best. The prosthetic prescription should entail information on the interface design/suspension method, the control system (external power, body power, etc.), the wrist features, and the appropriate terminal device(s).

Active prosthetic users should be prescribed at least one alternative device to guard against loss of function, should the primary prosthesis need repairs.

Current state of the science for externally powered transhumeral prostheses include options for only four powered degrees of freedom. These include elbow flexion/extension, wrist rotation, terminal device open/close, and thumb opposition.

The lack of sufficient, intuitive, control inputs is the most severe limiting factor to the advancement of powered upper limb prosthetic designs. Surgical advancements, such as TMR, and research into alternative inputs and control strategies, such as with the Defense Advanced Research Project Agency (DARPA) Revolutionizing Prosthetics Program, are paving the way toward improving the powered capabilities of externally powered prosthesis and developing new and intuitive ways for the user to control complex prosthetic movements.

REFERENCES

1. Daly WK. Elbow disarticulation and transhumeral amputation: prosthetic management. In: Smith DG, Michael JW, Bowker JH. Atlas of Amputations and Limb Deficiencies—Surgical, Prosthetic and Rehabilitation Principles, 3rd ed. *American Academy of Orthopedic Surgeons*, 2004:243–249.
2. Sensinger J, Pasquina PF, Kuiken T. The future of artificial limbs. In: Pasquina PF, Cooper RA. Textbooks of Military Medicine: Care of the

Combat Amputee. *The Office of the Surgeon General at TMM Publications*, 2009:721–730.

3. Lipshutz RD, Miller LA, Stubblefield KA, et al. Transhumeral level fitting and outcomes following targeted hyper-reinnervation nerve transfer surgery. From "MEC '05 Integrating Prosthetics and Medicine," Proceedings of the 2005 MyoElectric Controls/Powered Prosthetics Symposium, Fredericton, New Brunswick, Canada, August 17–19, 2005.
4. Kuiken TA, Li G, Lock BA, et al. Targeted muscle reinnervation for real-time myoelectric control of multifunction artificial arms. *JAMA*. 2009;301(6):619–628.
5. Resnik L, Meucci MR, Fantini C, et al. Advanced upper limb prosthetic devices: Implications for upper limb prosthetic rehabilitation. *Arch Phys Med Rehabil*. 2012:93:710–717.

RESOURCES

Meier RH, Atkins DJ. Functional Restoration of Adults and Children with Upper Extremity Amputation. *Demos Medical*, 2004.

Muzumdar A. Powered Upper Limb Prostheses—Control, Implementation and Clinical Application. *Springer-Verlag Berlin Heidelberg*, 2004.

Pasquina PF, Cooper RA. Textbooks of Military Medicine: Care of the Combat Amputee. *The Office of the Surgeon General at TMM Publications*, 2009.

Smith DG, Michael JW, Bowker JH. Atlas of Amputations and Limb Deficiencies—Surgical, Prosthetic and Rehabilitation Principles, 3rd ed. *American Academy of Orthopedic Surgeons*, 2004.

ADDITIONAL INFORMATION

- Website with general information about orthotics and prosthetics: http://www.oandp.com
- American Academy of Orthotists and Prosthetists: www.oandp.org
- Otto Bock—(manufacturer of many upper extremity prosthetic components including the Michelangelo hand): http://ottobockus.com/cps/rde/xchg/ob_us_en/hs.xsl/4713.html
- Motion Control—(manufacturer of externally powered prosthetic components): http://www.utaharm.com/index.php
- Liberating Technologies—(manufacturer of upper extremity prosthetic components): http://liberatingtechnologies.com/
- TRS—(manufacturer of body powered and specialty prosthetic components): http://www.oandp.com/products/trs/
- Texas Assistive Devices—(manufacturer of upper limb prosthetic components): http://n-abler.org/

- Touch Bionics—(manufacturer of the I-Limb hand): http://www.touchbionics.com/
- RSL Steeper—(manufacturer of upper extremity prosthetic components including the Bebionic hand): http://bebionic.com/
- http://dukespace.lib.duke.edu/dspace/bitstream/handle/10161/4752/68%20Schulz.pdf?sequence=1 – (First Experiences with the Vincent Hand)
- http://upperlimbprosthetics.info/
- http://arm-amp.com

18

Shoulder Disarticulation and Forequarter Amputation

Allison Hickman

Shoulder disarticulation and interscapulothoracic disarticulation (forequarter) represent the two most proximal arm amputation levels. Surgical disarticulation of the shoulder involves transection through the shoulder joint (sparing the scapular glenoid and scapulo-clavicular articulation). Amputations through the proximal humerus, sparing the humeral head, are treated as shoulder disarticulations. When possible, the primary advantage of retaining the humeral head is cosmesis. A forequarter amputation involves removing the entire shoulder girdle including the scapula and all or part of the clavicle. Surgical sparing of at least part of the clavicle is ideal in that it can continue to provide an anchor point for the pectoralis muscles. It should be noted that forequarter amputations are typically considered a limb salvage and lifesaving procedure to prevent scapular tumors from invading the chest wall [1]. As such, these patients often have the additional medical and psychological challenge of surviving a grave cancer diagnosis and the associated treatments prior to surgical intervention.

Fortunately, upper extremity amputation at the level of the shoulder disarticulation and forequarter amputation occur much less commonly than amputations at other levels. As mentioned above, the majority of these amputations are undertaken to remove a malignancy. In fact, only around 3% of traumatic amputations occur at this proximal level [2]. The proximal humerus is the third most common site for osteosarcoma and is the most common primary malignancy of the proximal humerus. In the scapula, chondrosarcoma and Ewing's sarcoma are the most common [3].

As would be expected, patients with these amputation levels are extremely difficult to fit with not only a functional prosthesis, but one that will be practical to use, even if intermittently. This is due to the extreme complexity and range of motion of the shoulder, elbow, wrist, and hand articulations. Added to this is the challenge of comfortable suspension to the body. For these reasons and many other individual reasons, patients with these levels of amputation often prefer to live without a prosthesis or alternately use an ultra lightweight passive cosmetic prosthesis [4–5]. There are no generalities when determining which patients will successfully integrate a complete upper limb prosthesis into their lives. As with any prosthesis, a multitude of patient and non-patient driven factors will influence desire, use, and tolerance of the device.

Terminal devices, wrist, and elbow components used in shoulder disarticulation and forequarter amputations do not vary greatly from, and usually are identical to, those used for patients with transhumeral or transradial amputation levels. For a review of prosthetic wrist and elbow component options, please see the chapters on transradial and transhumeral amputation. A shoulder unit and more complex suspension is needed for this level, and these components add a significant level of complexity to suspension and control of the prosthesis. More importantly, these components add weight and increase the potential for shear and pressure that can lead to skin breakdown and dermatitis caused by excess moisture and decreased ventilation of perspiration prone areas such as the axilla.

Similar to more distal amputations, patients with shoulder disarticulation or forequarter amputations have four general options for the type of prosthesis to be used, each with distinct advantages and disadvantages. These include a passive non-functional prosthesis, a passive functional prosthesis, a body (cable) powered prosthesis, an externally powered prosthesis (for example, myoelectric), or a hybrid that involves mixing body-powered and externally powered components to best meet the functional and aesthetic desires of the patient.

PASSIVE NON-FUNCTIONAL PROSTHESIS

A passive non-functional prosthesis is generally made of lightweight foam covered with polyvinyl chloride (PVC) or silicone and serves primarily to create the illusion of an intact limb. This can be especially important with amputation at the shoulder and forequarter levels to allow appropriate clothing fit and appearance. Maintenance is minimal, but depending on the material used, keeping the passive prosthesis clean can be an issue. Cost also varies greatly and depends on the material used and also the detail ascribed to the limb. Modern devices are usually fabricated of urethanes or similar synthetics with rigidity supplied by graphite, light metals, or semi-rigid thermoplastics when needed [6]. For an entirely passive prosthesis, the arm hangs from a fitted shoulder cap, and the elbow is simple and non-functional but can articulate so that it can be passively positioned by the sound limb. The hand can be contoured, painted, and textured to bear a striking resemblance to the sound limb. However, customization and use of specialized materials can not only increase the cost of the prosthesis but also make it more susceptible to damage and less resistant to everyday wear and tear.

PASSIVE FUNCTIONAL PROSTHESIS

A passive functional prosthesis can have any number of passive articulating joints that have manual lock/unlock mechanisms that can be used to place the limb in various positions using the sound limb or even a stationary object. A shoulder unit with this function could also be set to swing freely to simulate the normal arc of motion during gait. An elbow unit of this type can be used for carrying objects that are bulky or heavy enough to require two arms or for carrying a bag or purse to free up the sound limb. A passive wrist joint can operate with a manual lock or by friction depending on the needs of the amputee. As the name implies, these limbs provide minimal functionality, though they can be used to aid in balancing or pushing an object, or to secure an object between the prosthesis and the body.

BODY-POWERED PROSTHESES

Body-powered prostheses (using cables and pulleys) are typically of moderate cost and weight. Of all the prosthetic types above, they are typically the most durable and do tend to provide good sensory feedback to the residual limb and/or tissues. However, they can be bulky and therefore less cosmetically pleasing, especially when used to control several functional components as would be needed with this level of amputation. Also, operation of this type of prosthesis requires the ability for gross limb movement and torque generation. These movement patterns, such as shoulder flexion/extension/elevation and scapular retraction/elevation/rotation, may no longer be possible in the ipsilateral limb after shoulder or forequarter amputation. In such cases, movement patterns of the intact contralateral limb can be used, but this is generally not practical or well accepted by the patient. In general, due to suspension difficulty and lack of residual functional movement to operate the cables, body-powered prostheses are not used for forequarter amputees. Possible configurations for use in shoulder disarticulation are explained in the following section on harnessing and suspension.

EXTERNALLY POWERED PROSTHESES

Externally powered (myoelectric or switch control) prostheses for the upper extremity are becoming increasingly more sophisticated in their functionality with efforts to maximize utility while reducing weight. Myoelectric controlled prosthesis depend on the patient's ability to contract residual muscles. These contractions create an electrical signal that is detected by surface electrodes and transmitted to motors that drive the functional component(s). When physiologic muscle pairs are available (flexion/extension and pronation/supination), a two-site/two-function system can be used. This is the easiest setup to control in that one muscle action produces a distinct movement of the device. This system, however, is not possible for patients with shoulder or forequarter amputation due to the limited number of ipsilateral muscle control sites. In this case, a one-site/two-function or sequential/multistate controller can be used and the pectoralis muscle is most often used. With the former setup, one electrode controls both functions of a paired activity (flexion/extension) and depends on graded (proportional) contraction of the control muscle (a weak contraction closes the device and a strong contraction opens it). The latter configuration allows for the control of several functions using a single electrode pair. This requires the control function of the electrodes to be switched from one function to another. This can be accomplished by a brief co-contraction of the muscle (an option not available in shoulder or forequarter amputation) or by activation of a manual switch. Many contemporary myoelectric prostheses operate using graded or proportional control so that the force generated or the speed of movement of the functional component varies with the intensity of the muscle contraction.

Alternatively, a switch-control externally powered prosthesis is an option when adequate myoelectric control sites are not available or when the patient has difficultly mastering control of a myoelectric unit. As the name implies, small switches, instead of muscle signals, are used to operate the electric motors of the functional component. Most commonly these switches are integrated into the socket or sometimes into the suspension harness. The switch is activated by compression with the residual limb, or against a bony prominence, or by a pull on the suspension harness similar to the motion to activate a body-powered prosthesis. Advantages of externally powered devices can include greater torque generation at both proximal and terminal components as well as improved cosmesis. Disadvantages include increasing weight as more functional components/movements are added, sensory feedback is often less or non-existent compared to that of a body-powered unit, maintenance of the unit (including components and battery charging), and cost.

HYBRID UPPER EXTREMITY PROSTHESIS

A hybrid upper extremity prosthesis, as the name implies, uses any combination of cosmetic, body and externally powered components. This configuration is the most practical for a shoulder disarticulation or forequarter amputee if and when they choose to wear a functional over a passive prosthesis. Typically the shoulder unit is a passive, manual, or switch locking device that can be placed at various angles by the sound limb (Figure 18.1). A shoulder disarticulation amputee could then use a passive locking, body driven or myoelectric elbow paired with passive locking or friction controlled wrist unit, and a cable driven or myoelectric terminal device depending on available control motions (cable) and/or muscles (myoelectric). For the forequarter amputee, use of bi-scapular motion is not possible and as such the use of body-powered devices is generally difficult if not impossible, and therefore not well accepted. If a myoelectric terminal device is desired it is usually paired with a manual locking shoulder and elbow unit and a manual locking or friction controlled wrist. The ipsilateral pectoral muscles can be used to control the terminal device. However, as stated previously, increasing the number of functional components adds weight, which adds the need for increased strapping and suspension and a wider thorax footprint for the socket.

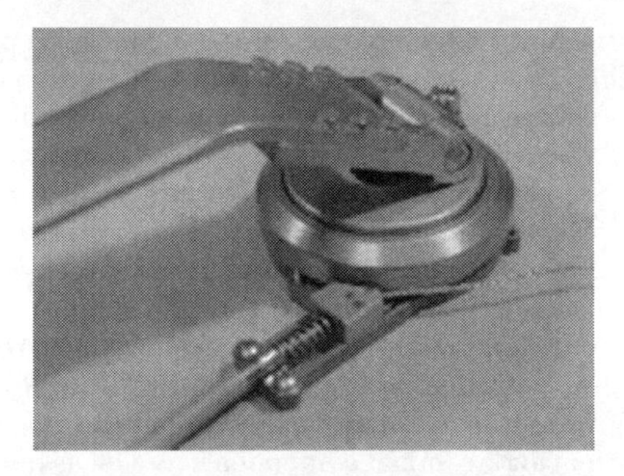

Figure 18.1 LTI locking shoulder joint, body-powered shoulder.
Courtesy of Liberating Technologies Inc. (LTI).

In general, regardless of functionality and control of the shoulder component, one overriding functional deficiency of both body-powered and externally powered devices for patients with shoulder disarticulation and forequarter amputation is the inability to functionally operate the shoulder unit above roughly 90° of abduction or flexion. An exception to this is with advanced technology that is not currently commercially available. These devices are described at the end of this chapter.

PROSTHETIC SUSPENSION AND HARNESSING FOR PATIENTS WITH SHOULDER DISARTICULATION OR FOREQUARTER AMPUTATION

Suspension of an upper extremity prosthetic for shoulder or forequarter amputation requires extending the prosthesis onto the thorax using a casted thermoplastic socket with variable coverage and strapping configurations depending on the needs of the amputee. It is often a struggle to find a suspension modality that provides a snug fit and allows for functional use of the prosthetic components while at the same time being comfortable enough for extended wear and allowing the amputee to don/doff the prosthesis as independently as possible. Indeed this combination of variables, not to mention the time and effort it takes to use and maintain a prosthesis with high level arm amputation, relegates the vast majority of these amputees to elect for a lightweight passive prosthesis or no prosthesis at all. At this amputation level a simple shoulder cap is an option and can be molded from lightweight flexible foam to have a similar shape and contour of the contralateral shoulder. The amputee can then decide whether or not to suspend a passive arm from this cap to further fill out clothing and provide a more natural appearance.

Even a lightweight cosmetic shoulder cap, however, requires suspension. This has traditionally been achieved with the use of web or nylon straps, typically with a hook and loop component to facilitate independent donning/doffing. The cap is placed over the residual shoulder structure and the strap (originating from the anterior and posterior portions of the cap) is looped under the contralateral axilla. Alternatively, adhesive pads can be applied to the cap which, depending on the patient, may eliminate the need for straps and can also minimize movement and slippage of the cap.

Naturally, as the weight of the prosthesis increases with the addition of more functional shoulder, elbow, wrist, and hand units, the robustness of the suspension must also increase. For most amputees, this is the primary limiting factor for regular use of the prosthetic device.

As mentioned previously, manually locking functional units can be used at the shoulder, elbow, and wrist; however these are not ideal in that they require occupying the sound limb for engagement of the locking mechanism. The chin is sometimes used to operate a manual switch; however this movement can be awkward and unnatural and therefore not well accepted by most amputees. This is where creative harnessing for body controlled units can occasionally be useful. The perineal strap functions on the basis of relative displacement between the shoulders and the pelvis but, for obvious reasons, this can be uncomfortable and is not well accepted by most amputees. The more commonly used chest and waist strap combinations are typically better tolerated. Men have more options when it comes to harnessing and operating a arm prosthesis in this fashion due to the ability to easily place a strap across the chest and, generally, a broader chest to allow for increased excursion and subsequent movement range of the functional unit. For women, creative solutions integrating a brazier have been devised. Men and larger women may also have a small advantage in operating these systems in that movement of the unit depends on excursion of the control source, as such, the greater the distance of excursion, the more the movement that can be generated.

Dual Control Harness

The most commonly used dual control harness for a male with shoulder disarticulation involves scapular abduction for dual control of forearm flexion at the elbow and terminal device operation (open/close) that occurs as a single motion when the elbow is unlocked. When the elbow is locked, scapular motion controls only the terminal device. The elbow lock is managed by the elevation of the shoulder on the ipsilateral side. This is controlled by a chest strap that attaches to the front of the shoulder cap, passes under the axilla on the contralateral side, crosses the back at the mid-scapular level, and then attaches to the control cable positioned on the back of the shoulder cap. An elastic strap extends from the top of the shoulder cap, proceeds medially across the back, and attaches to the chest strap just lateral of the spine towards the sound limb. With this configuration, bi-scapular abduction activates a terminal device. This is typically a voluntary opening hook or greifer. The elbow lock is operated by shoulder elevation by linking the elbow control cable to a waist strap placed just below the thoracic cage for an anchor point. This configuration is typically the easiest to learn and use.

Another commonly used dual control shoulder disarticulation harness system also uses bi-scapular abduction for dual control of elbow flexion and the terminal device, but the elbow lock is controlled by forward flexion of the contralateral shoulder. Elbow flexion and opening/closing of the terminal device are controlled in the same manner as in the previous configuration. To control the elbow lock with this harness, the contralateral shoulder has a webbing "saddle" with a strap that runs from the superior part of that webbing, across the back (above the scapular abduction strap), and attached to the elbow control cable through the back of the shoulder cap. Though this system eliminates the need for a waist strap, it does add more complicated harnessing about the shoulders. Also, the elbow lock/unlock could be inadvertently activated while the elbow is being flexed and/or the terminal device is being operated.

Triple Control Shoulder Disarticulation Harness

For a triple control shoulder disarticulation harness, three functions are provided by three control sources. The typical configuration utilizes scapular abduction for forearm flexion, shoulder shrug on the contralateral side for control of the terminal device, and elevation of the shoulder on the amputated side to operate the elbow lock. The harnessing configuration is a hybrid of the previous two and requires the use of a waist strap and a webbing saddle on the contralateral shoulder with the addition of a control strap across the back, at about the level of the spinous process of the seventh cervical vertebra, to the posterior/superior shoulder cap to operate the terminal device.

Though this configuration requires more harnessing than the dual control system it does offer certain advantages. The separation of terminal device operation from forearm flexion can improve control of prehension. This is because during forearm flexion (scapular abduction) no concurrent action takes place at the terminal device as in the dual control system. Additionally, since the elbow lock is operated by an independent motion (ipsilateral shoulder elevation) there is less chance of inadvertently activating this component.

For most women with shoulder disarticulation, the chest strap will not be a viable option. To compensate for this, the webbing strap that wraps around the torso can be incorporated into the bottom part of a brazier using clips or D-ring attachments so that the garment can be easily separated from the harness for regular cleaning. Using this method, a dual or triple control system can be used with minimal other strapping modifications to the male configurations.

Unfortunately, long term use of a body-powered prostheses can cause or accelerate the progression of debilitating shoulder overuse issues of both the amputated and the sound limb. The amputee can also develop anterior muscle strains and imbalances, and also nerve entrapment issues from socket pressure on the amputated side and strapping pressure on the contralateral axilla [7].

MYOELECTRIC CONTROLS FOR PATIENTS WITH SHOULDER DISARTICULATION OR FOREQUARTER AMPUTATION

For the shoulder disarticulation amputee, both myoelectric and switch activated controls could be used to operate a prosthesis. For those with forequarter amputation, myoelectric control using the pectoralis muscle is the primary option when an externally powered or hybrid prosthesis is desired. Currently available myoelectric control devices for operating a complete upper extremity prosthesis offer several advantages over body controlled devices. This includes at least partially eliminating the need to use the sound limb to position or lock a functional unit in place. Removing cable control also makes the prosthesis less bulky and allows for internalization of components within an exoskeleton to provide a more natural appearance of the limb. And depending on the components and ability of the amputee, movement speed and unit force actuation can be increased. Lastly, since battery powered motors are used to drive the components, the need for exaggerated or non-anatomic movement patterns is for the most part eliminated, thus decreasing the potential for muscle strain and overuse injuries. Disadvantages include increased weight of prosthesis, which in turn increases the bulk and complexity of suspension, significant increase in cost and maintenance, and decrease in durability. Lastly, externally powered devices currently are not well suited for heavy lifting or manual labor in dirty or wet environments.

As an alternative to a myoelectric device, patients with shoulder disarticulation may be able to use the anterior and posterior bony prominences of the glenoid rim, prominent acromion, or a preserved humeral head to activate pressure switches embedded in the shoulder cap of the prosthetic. These switches could be used to power supination/pronation of an externally powered elbow unit and/or to open and close a hand unit in a graded or all-or-nothing maneuver. A multistate touch control could also be used allowing the patient to activate the elbow or the terminal device but each unit control would be independent requiring the patient to switch back and forth between the components.

Until recently, myoelectric electrodes placed over the pectoral muscle served as the primary basis for the control of a complete upper arm prosthesis. Though this was a significant advancement, operation of the limb required the amputee to learn physiologically unrelated motor activation patterns using the graded or sequential activation of the pectoralis to operate the limb. Also, to limit the complexity of pectoral activation, the number/type of functional movement is limited. Generally, only one degree of freedom (movement in one plane/direction) can be controlled at a time. With time and practice, however, the appropriately selected and motivated amputee can use this technology very well.

In efforts to improve the functionality of surface electrodes placed over the pectoral muscle, targeted muscle re-innervation (TMR) was first introduced by Lipshutz and colleagues in 2005 [8]. The concept is to control function in the prosthesis as would be done in the natural arm, therefore making the device more natural and easier to use. Assuming there is no damage to the remaining nerves of the brachial plexus, this is accomplished by surgically transferring the musculocutaneous, median, radial, and ulnar nerves to separate areas of the ipsilateral pectoralis muscle. Once healed, socket integrated myoelectrodes are strategically placed over the re-innervated muscle segments and their signals coordinated with individual but microprocessor linked arm control units (Figure 18.2). Ideally, this would allow for elbow flexion (musculocutaneous), hand and wrist flexion (median), extension of the elbow, wrist and hand (radial) and wrist flexion, and finger abduction (ulnar) of the prosthesis. With successful

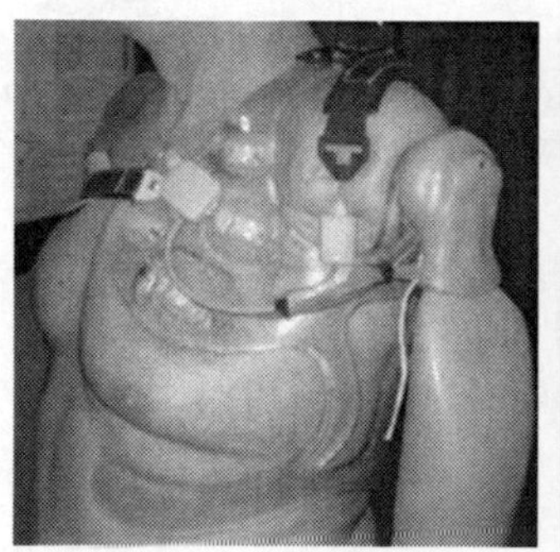
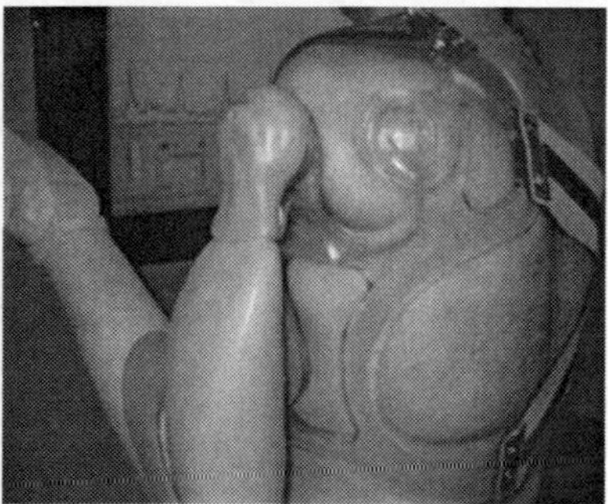

Figure 18.2 Targeted muscle re-innervation patient.
***Source*: From Advanced Arm Dynamics, Redondo Beach, CA. Used with permission.**

re-innervation and rehabilitation, and with the use of advanced upper extremity prosthetics (see the next section) the amputee can potentially operate myoelectric site signals allowing varying degrees of simultaneous coordination of shoulder, elbow, wrist, and hand movement. The complexity and efficiency of the movement will depend on the amputee's ability to control the device and the technological capability of the prosthesis itself.

ADVANCED TECHNOLOGIES FOR COMPLETE UPPER EXTREMITY PROSTHESES AND CONTROL

Though it is unlikely that a prosthetic device will ever mirror the functional complexity and cosmetic and dynamic aesthetics of a natural arm, advanced robotic systems continue to push the envelope in efforts to provide upper extremity amputees with more realistic options. These advances include the ability to control a shoulder unit and distal units simultaneously during overhead activities, increased speed and accuracy of prosthetic movements, and tactile methods such as vibration and LED sensors to synthesize sensory inputs. With limited exceptions, most current myoelectric full arm prostheses for those with shoulder disarticulation or forequarter amputation are experimental and/or part of highly selective clinical trials. Defense Advanced Research Projects Agency (DARPA), in efforts to develop advanced prostheses for U.S. military service members has helped fund the development of the DEKA arm and the Luke arm (DEKA Integrated Solutions Corporation), and the APL arm (Johns Hopkins

Applied Physics Lab). These are prototypes and not currently slated for mass production but their development and continued refinement will no doubt be integral to furthering advances in bio-prosthetic integration and control.

REFERENCES

1. Dillingham T, MacKenzie E. Limb amputation and limb deficiency: Epidemiology and recent trends in the United States. *South Med J*. 2002 Aug;95(8):875–883.
2. Anderson-Ranberg F, Ebskov B. Major upper extremity amputation in Denmark. *Acta Orthop Scand*. 1988;59:321.
3. Cuccurullo S. *Physical Medicine and Rehabilitation Board Review*, Demos Medical Publishing; 2004.
4. Roeschlein RA, Domholdt E. Factors related to successful upper extremity prosthetic use. *Prosthet Orthot Int*. 1989;13:14–18.
5. Fraser CM. An evaluation of the use made of cosmetic and functional prostheses by unilateral upper limb amputees. *Prosthet Orthot Int*. 1998;22:216–223.
6. *Rockwood and Matsen's the Shoulder: Expert Consult*, Elsevier Health Sciences; 2009.
7. Jones LE, Davidson JH. Save that arm: A study of problems in the remaining arm of unilateral upper limb amputees. *Prosthet Orthot Int*. 1999;23:55–58.
8. Lipshutz RD, Kuiken TA, Miller LA, Dumanian GA, Stubblefield KA. Shoulder disarticulation externally powered prosthetic fitting following targeted muscle reinnervation for improved myoelectric control. *J Prosth Orth*. 2006;18(2):28–34.

19

Normal Human Gait

Joseph Webster

Bipedal ambulation is a unique and fascinating human activity. While normal human gait can appear simple, effortless, and even mundane to the casual observer, it is actually a complex phenomenon and its understanding requires a solid appreciation of biomechanical terminology and principles. Understanding normal gait is essential to the evaluation and management of abnormal gait patterns. This is especially true for gait deviations seen in individuals with amputations who ambulate with the use of prosthetic limbs.

Although there are a range of gait "differences" that can be considered "within normal limits," this chapter will cover previously accepted and reported normal gait parameters and definitions. This chapter includes the following aspects of normal gait: terminology and definitions, determinants of normal gait, sagittal plane kinematic and kinetic analysis, and EMG (muscle) activity.

GENERAL TERMINOLOGY AND DEFINITIONS

Kinesiology—The analysis and description of motion.

Kinematics—The description of human motion without regard to the forces producing or opposing the movement.

Kinetics—The study of the forces producing motion or maintaining equilibrium.

Vector—A representation of a force graphically in terms of its magnitude, line of application, direction, and point of application.

Ground Reaction Force (GRF)—In weight-bearing, the forces that act on the body as a result of its interaction with the ground. The GRFs are equal and opposite to the force the body is applying to the ground.

Ground Reaction Force Vector (GRFV)—The vector representation of the GRF.

Moment or Torque—The measure of the tendency of a force to produce rotation about a point or axis. Torque applies to rotatory motion and is the product of a force applied perpendicular to a lever arm and the distance of the force application from the axis of motion.

Moment Arm—The shortest distance from an action line (the line through which a force acts) and the axis of motion.

Thus, Torque = Force × Moment Arm

Center of Mass/Gravity (COG)—In quiet standing, the COG is considered to be located just anterior to the second sacral vertebra.

Center of Pressure—The origin or point of application of the GRF on the body. It is the theoretical point where the force is considered to act.

Observational Gait Analysis—The visual observation of gait that occurs in real time as the person ambulates. Observational gait analysis does not rely on any other measures or tools and only addresses the motion and movement that is occurring during ambulation.

Quantitative Gait Analysis—This analysis is performed in a formal gait lab setting and provides quantitative information regarding gait which can include kinematics, kinetics, muscle activity, and energetics (analysis of metabolic and mechanical energy).

Gait Cycle Terminology (Figures 19.1 and 19.2)

Stride—The basic unit of gait which occurs between initial contact of a limb (reference limb) and the subsequent initial contact of that same limb.

Stride Length—The distance traveled during one gait cycle or stride.

Step Length—The distance traveled during one step (initial contact to end of preswing on the same limb).

Step Width—The distance between the center of the feet during the double limb support portion of the gait cycle when both feet are in contact with the ground. This distance is normally 7 to 8 cm.

Cadence—The number of steps taken in a given period of time (commonly expressed as steps per minute). Average cadence during normal human ambulation is 80 to 110 steps/minute. This corresponds to an average walking speed of 60 to 80 m/minute.

Stance Phase—The portion of the gait cycle during which the reference limb is in contact with the ground. During normal walking, this portion accounts for approximately 60% of the gait cycle. Stance phase includes initial contact, loading response, midstance, terminal stance, and preswing.

Swing Phase—The portion of the gait cycle during which the reference limb in not in contact with the ground. During normal walking, this portion accounts for approximately 40% of the gait cycle. Swing phase includes initial swing, midswing, and terminal swing.

Single Limb Support—The portion of the gait cycle during which only one limb is in contact with the ground. During normal gait, this segment accounts for 40% of the total gait cycle. Single limb support includes midstance and terminal stance.

Double Limb Support—The portion of the gait cycle during which two limbs are in contact with the ground. During normal gait, this portion accounts for 20% of the gait cycle. Double limb support includes three different components of the gait cycle: initial contact, loading response, and preswing.

Functional Tasks of Normal Gait—The functional tasks of normal human gait are typically described as weight acceptance, single limb support, and limb advancement.

Traditional Gait Terminology—This terminology is no longer the preferred terminology used in the description of gait. This terminology generally describes isolated points in time during the gait cycle rather than periods of time. This terminology is included in this chapter as a historical reference and because these terms are also still occasionally used/heard in the clinical setting.

Stance Phase

1. Heel Strike—The point when the heel makes contact with the ground.
2. Foot Flat—The point when the sole of the foot makes contact with the ground.
3. Midstance—The point at which full body weight is taken by the limb.
4. Heel Off—The point after midstance when the heel leaves the ground.
5. Toe Off—The last point of stance phase when the toe loses contact with the ground.

Swing Phase

1. Acceleration—The time period from toe off to midswing.
2. Midswing—The mid-portion of swing phase when the limb is directly below the body.
3. Deceleration—The last portion of swing phase when the limb is slowing down in preparation for heel strike.

Rancho Los Amigos Gait Terminology

The Rancho Los Amigos Gait Terminology is the preferred terminology to be used in the description of gait.

Stance Phase

1. Initial Contact—Point in time when foot comes in contact with the ground.
2. Loading Response (LR)—Initial contact to the time when the contralateral foot leaves the ground.
3. Midstance (MSt)—From the time the contralateral foot leaves the ground to the time that the ipsilateral heel leaves the ground.
4. Terminal Stance (TSt)—From the time that the ipsilateral heel leaves the ground to the time of contralateral foot's initial contact with the ground.
5. Preswing (PSw)—From the time of the contralateral foot's initial contact with the ground to the time that the ipsilateral foot leaves the ground.

Swing Phase

- Initial Swing (ISw)—The time from when the foot leaves the ground to the ipsilateral foot alignment with the contralateral ankle.
- Midswing (MSw)—The time from ankle and foot alignment to the swing leg tibia becoming vertical.
- Terminal Swing (TSw)—The time from the tibia reaching a vertical position to initial contact of the swing foot with the ground.

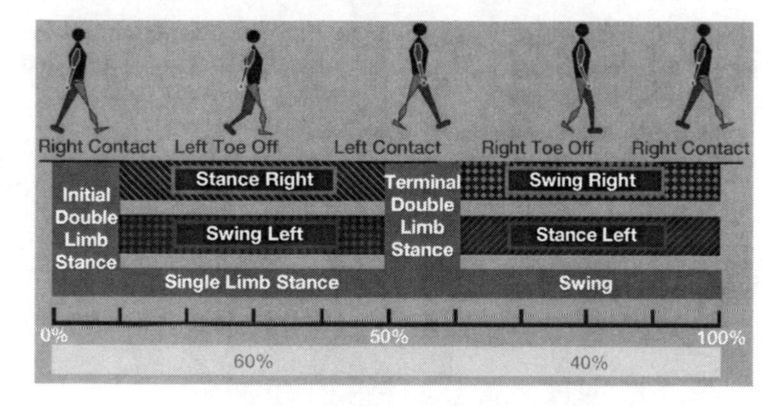

Figure 19.1 Gait cycle phases and timing.

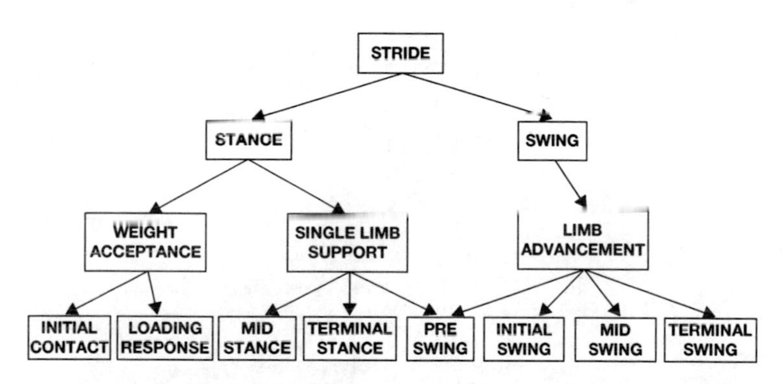

Figure 19.2 Gait cycle terminology and functional tasks.

DETERMINANTS OF GAIT

The six determinants of gait were originally described by Saunders and Inman in 1953 [1]. These determinants were used to describe strategies by which gait is made more efficient through minimizing the movement of the COG. As a person ambulates with a normal gait pattern, the COG follows a smooth, sinusoidal path in the frontal, transverse, and sagittal planes. The actual COG displacement is approximately 5 cm (2 inches) in each plane during normal gait. Descriptions of the six determinants of gait that minimize movement of the COG vary in different references and have been revised over time [2–4]. In general, the determinants can be classified into those occurring at the level of the pelvis and those occurring in the foot and ankle mechanisms (Figures 19.3–19.5).

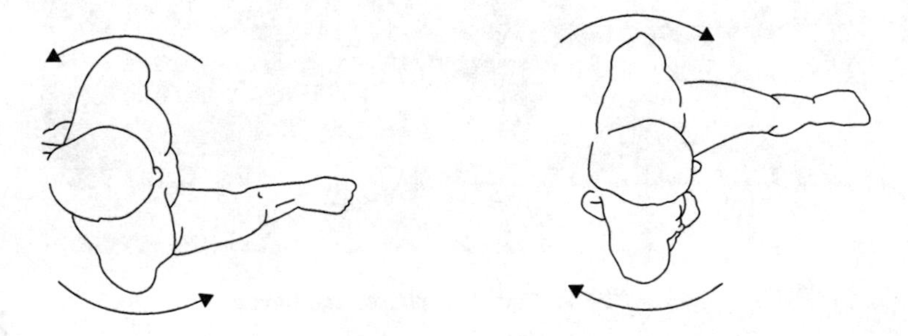

Figure 19.3 Pelvic rotation.

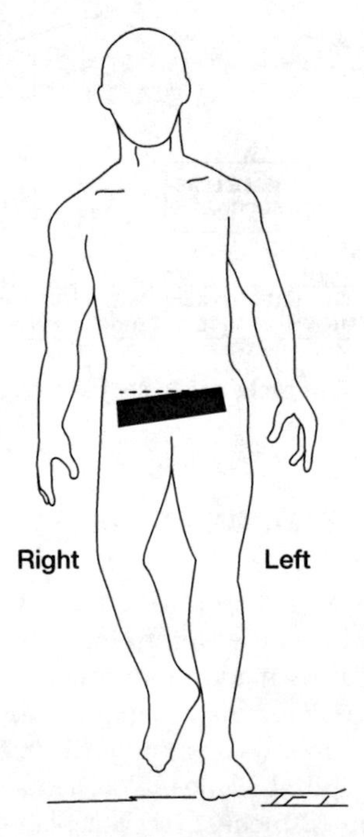

Figure 19.4 Pelvic tilt in the frontal plane.

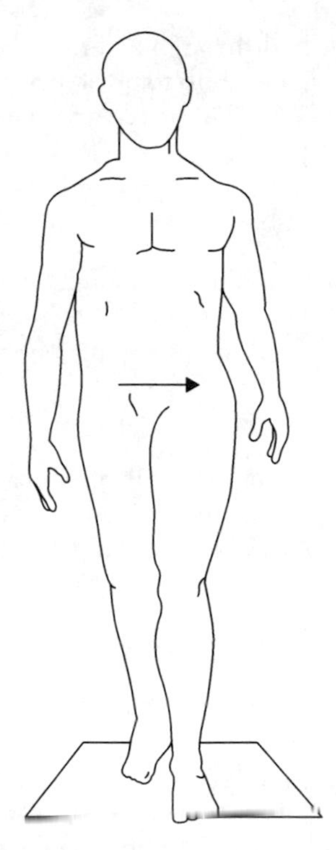

Figure 19.5 Lateral pelvic displacement.

The determinants can be further classified into the following:

1. Pelvic rotation in the horizontal plane
2. Pelvic tilt in the frontal plane
3. Lateral displacement of the pelvis
4. Early knee flexion
5. Foot and ankle mechanisms
6. Late knee flexion

ROCKERS: PIVOT POINTS DURING STANCE

During the stance phase of gait, the body needs to continue forward progression while the foot remains in stationary contact with the ground. Facilitating the body's progression forward requires a balance between progression and maintaining stability of the stance limb. This is accomplished through a series of rockers in the ankle and foot that allow the stance limb to pivot forward sequentially while the foot remains stationary. These rockers have been divided into four key areas by Perry [4].

Heel Rocker

Following initial contact and during loading response, the heel serves as the pivot point and the foot moves from a neutral position to 10° of plantarflexion.

Ankle Rocker

At the beginning of midstance, the pivot point/fulcrum point moves from the heel to the ankle. During midstance, the tibia and more proximal aspect of the limb, rotate forward at the ankle along the line of progression. This allows advancement of the stance limb and the body.

Forefoot Rocker

As the limb moves into terminal stance and the heel comes off the ground, the pivot point shifts to the forefoot and the rounded contour of the metatarsal heads. During this period, forward progression is accelerated as the body weight falls beyond the area of foot support.

Toe Rocker

In the final stages of stance phase, during preswing, the toe serves as the final pivot point for the body's continued forward movement and transition into swing phase.

KINEMATICS

Sagittal Plane Kinematics

Description of the motion that occurs at the hip, knee, and ankle during normal human gait in the sagittal plane; see Figure 19.6 [3–6].

Hip

The hip begins the gait cycle in approximately 30° of flexion at the time of initial contact. The hip is gradually extending throughout stance phase. The hip reaches a maximum extension of 10° at the end

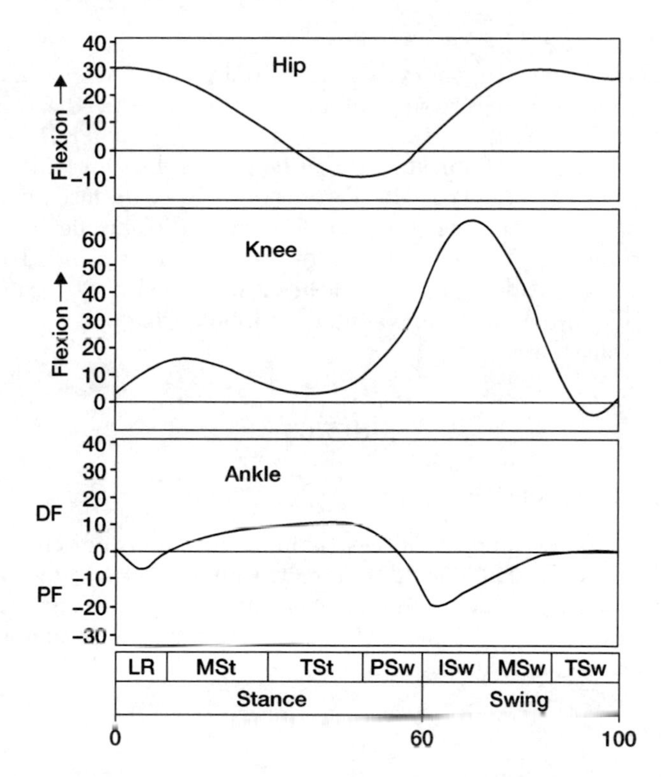

Figure 19.6 The hip, knee, and ankle ROM during gait.

of terminal stance. At the beginning of preswing, the hip begins to flex before the foot leaves contact with the ground. The hip gradually flexes during the swing phase reaching peak flexion of just over 30° just prior to initial contact.

Knee

The knee begins the gait cycle with approximately 5° of flexion at initial contact. The knee flexes slightly during loading response from 10° to 15° of flexion. Once the limb is in single limb support at the beginning of midstance, the knee begins to extend and it reaches –5° of full extension before beginning a period of rapid knee flexion at the end of stance phase and into initial swing phase. During swing phase, the knee reaches a maximum flexion of approximately 60° during midswing before moving into a period of knee extension. The knee reaches full extension at the end of swing phase and begins to flex slightly just prior to initial contact.

Ankle

The ankle begins the gait cycle in a neutral position at the time of initial contact. There is rapid plantarflexion from 5° to 12° that occurs during the loading response. This period of plantarflexion is followed by a time of gradual dorsiflexion that continues through midstance and terminal stance. Peak dorsiflexion of 10° occurs just prior to preswing. During preswing, the ankle begins to plantarflex rapidly prior to the foot leaving contact with the floor. This plantarflexion continues into early swing and reaches a maximum of 20° prior to the ankle moving back into a neutral position during the remainder of the swing phase.

KINETICS

Sagittal Plane Kinetics

This is the description of forces (moments) that occur across the hip, knee, and ankle joints during gait. Kinetics can also take into consideration metabolic and mechanical energy. Because these forces are created when the limb is in contact with the ground, they are described only during the stance phase of the gait cycle; see Figure 19.7 [3–6].

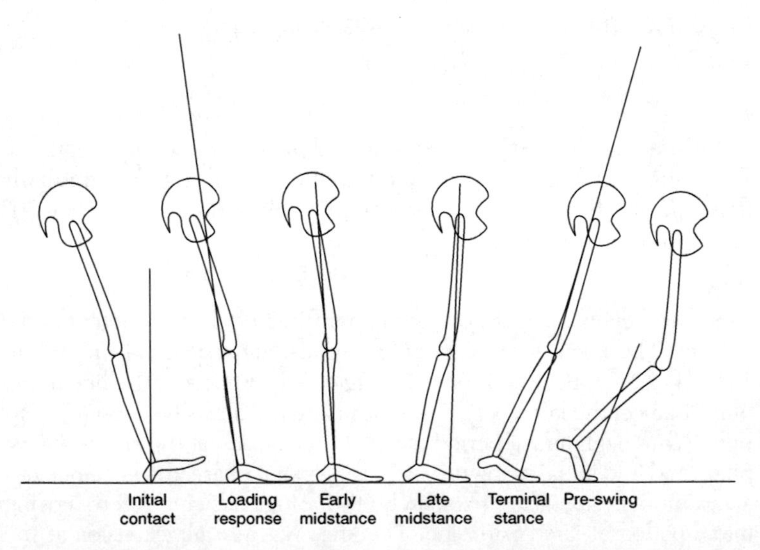

Figure 19.7 The GRF in relation to the lower limb joints during stance.

Hip

The GRF is initially anterior to the hip point of rotation which creates a flexion moment on the hip at initial contact and during the loading response. During midstance, as the tibia rotates forward, the hip moves anterior to the GRF creating an extension moment. This extension torque across the hip remains in place throughout the remainder of stance phase and active hip flexion is required to overcome this moment in late stance in order to initiate hip flexion.

Knee

At initial contact, the GRF is normally located anterior to the knee, but the GRF quickly moves posterior to the knee during the loading response which creates a flexion moment at the knee. This force is opposed by the quadriceps in order to keep the knee from collapsing. The knee flexion moment remains in place until terminal stance at which time the GRF moves back anterior to the knee. At the end of preswing, just prior to the foot leaving the ground, the period of rapid knee flexion begins and once the GRF moves posterior to the knee, the knee flexion moment that is created helps to facilitate this motion.

Ankle

The GRF is initially located posterior to the ankle at the time of initial contact which creates a plantarflexion moment at the ankle. During the loading response, the plantarflexion moment continues at the ankle and this moment has to be resisted by the ankle dorsiflexors to prevent foot drop. During midstance, the GRF moves anterior to the ankle and in terminal stance, there is a strong dorsiflexion moment at the ankle which must be opposed by the ankle plantarflexors in order to limit forward progression of the tibia. In preswing, a dorsiflexion moment remains at the ankle. Thus, ankle plantarflexion motion is created by concentric contraction of the ankle plantarflexors and this helps to propel the stance limb forward.

MUSCLE ACTIVITY/ELECTROMYOGRAPHIC ANALYSIS

EMG Muscle Activity

Pelvic and lower extremity muscles generate forces to produce movement, to resist GRFs, and to maintain equilibrium. The timing and extent of these muscle contractions as reported in the literature varies in different references [3–6]. The information included here is a synthesis of different references and is meant to provide a general description of the muscle activity that is occurring in the lower extremity to either produce or inhibit motion in the sagittal plane during dynamic gait. The muscle groups listed below are either active or inactive during different phases of the gait cycle. For the purpose of this text, only the gait cycle phase in which the muscle group is active is listed.

Hip Extensors

1. Late swing—Concentric contraction to rotate the thigh posteriorly and to stabilize the limb in preparation for weight-bearing in stance phase.
2. Early stance—Concentric or isometric contraction to control hip and knee flexion and stabilize the limb.

Hip Flexors

1. Late stance phase—Eccentric contraction to slow and control posterior rotation (extension) of the thigh.
2. Swing phase—Concentric contraction to initiate hip flexion and accelerate the swing limb forward.

Knee Extensors

1. Initial contact and loading response—Eccentric contraction to control knee flexion and prevent knee buckling.
2. Late stance and early swing phase—Eccentric contraction to control collapse of the knee and prevent early heel rise.

Knee Flexors

1. Flexion and facilitate foot clearance in swing phase.
2. Late swing phase and early stance phase—Eccentric and isometric contraction to control knee extension and stabilize the limb prior to weight-bearing.

Ankle Dorsiflexors

1. Early stance phase—Eccentric contraction to control ankle plantarflexion in loading response.
2. Swing phase—Concentric contraction for ankle dorsiflexion and to facilitate foot clearance during swing phase.

Ankle Plantarflexors

1. Midstance phase—Eccentric contraction to control the ankle dorsiflexion moment and prevent excessive forward tibia rotation.
2. Terminal stance and preswing phase—Concentric contraction for push-off and acceleration of the swing limb.

REFERENCES

1. Saunders JB, Inman VT, Eberhart HD. The major determinants in normal and pathological gait. *J Bone Joint Surg Am.* 1953;35-A(3):543–558.
2. Della Croce U, Riley PO, Lelas JL, Kerrigan DC. A refined view of the determinants of gait. *Gait Posture.* 2001;14(2):79–84.
3. Waters RL, Mulroy S. The energy expenditure of normal and pathologic gait. *Gait Posture.* 1999;9(3):207–231.
4. Perry J, Burnfield JM. *Gait Analysis: Normal and Pathologic Function,* 2nd ed. SLACK Incorp; 2010.
5. Norkin CC, Levangie PK. *Joint Structure and Function: A Comprehensive Analysis.* 2nd ed. F.A. Davis Co; 1992.
6. Esqunazi A, Talaty M. Gait analysis: Technology and clinical applications. In: Braddom RL, ed. *Physical Medicine and Rehabilitation.* 4th ed. Elsevier Inc; 2011;99–117.

20

Gait Deviations After Limb Loss

Leif Nelson

A key to a successful rehabilitation prescription for a person with lower extremity limb loss is interpreting observational gait analysis, by using clinical evaluation findings. With few exceptions, the simplest strategy is to observe for symmetry or the lack thereof [1]. There are a few asymmetrical gait deviations that would historically be considered "normal" for this population [2,3], but with current prosthetic technologies that are available, improved symmetry is possible [4,5], particularly for the patient who is intrinsically motivated and has the proper physical therapy prescription [6].

Gait deviations have been classified in many different ways, but the key to diagnostically determining the cause stems from the point in the gait cycle the abnormality occurs, most grossly during swing or stance phase. Observational findings can lead to specific intervention prescription once they are coupled with a full evaluation of the patient with and without the prosthesis donned. Decreased walking speed, wider base of support, and decreased balance are typically common findings for persons with lower extremity limb loss [6–12], and mitigating causes should be investigated by the clinician. Knee flexion contractures for transtibial amputees and hip flexion and/or abduction contractures for transfemoral amputees are common, and all but guarantee that the patient will ambulate with an asymmetrical gait pattern. In addition, range of motion testing for the intact lower extremity is also crucial, especially in traumatic etiology, as this can be an overlooked root cause for a gait deviation. Manual muscle strength testing can also be a key to diagnosing the root of an abnormality that is observed during ambulation. Patient subjective feedback, along with hands-on assessment of socket fit, will be the final pieces of the puzzle in determining the cause of an asymmetrical gait pattern.

During your observational gait analysis, it is absolutely necessary to observe the patient ambulating in both the frontal and sagittal planes. This chapter will cover the most common gait deviations in persons with lower extremity limb loss, but be aware that additional comorbidities may lead to additional deviations, so always correlate observations with a complete physical evaluation.

The following gait deviations for patients with limb loss are from a career of clinical experience, and whenever possible evidence has been cited from other authors to substantiate the empirically based claims.

STANCE PHASE DEVIATIONS

Foot Slap on Prosthetic Side at Initial Contact

This deviation is less common today than many of the deviations that follow, grossly speaking, as there is a trend in prescribing non-articulating flex-foot style prosthetic feet for their benefits in lowering energy cost during ambulation [13]. There is, however, research that suggests, for the older population with limb loss secondary to vascular disease, an articulating ankle may be indicated to promote increased symmetry in gait [14]. Foot slap is typically caused by a worn-out or missing plantarflexion bumper on an articulating ankle prosthetic foot. If the patient achieves a true heel strike at initial contact, this deviation is facilitated by the ground-reaction force which is posterior to the ankle joint. This is best visualized in the sagittal plane.

Foot Rotation on Prosthetic Side at Heel Strike

Increased wear on the lateral aspect of the heel of proper footwear is typical, meaning weight at initial contact for anyone who ambulates with heel strike is posterior-lateral [15]. In the lower extremity limb loss population, if the prosthetic heel (cushion) is too hard, the foot will pivot at initial contact and loading response phases of gait, and lead to excessive toe-out or foot rotation on the prosthetic side. This will similarly occur if the plantar flexion bumper is too stiff.

An even more common cause of this would be poor socket fit on the residual limb. Rotation of the entire prosthesis can occur if transverse plane movement is not controlled by current socket fit. This loss of socket suspension will lead to observation of excessive toe-out. The intervention for this is typically patient education as to proper socket ply. As the day progresses, loss of limb volume is common, and thus the addition of residual limb socks can help maintain socket suspension. Alternately, excessive sock ply can also lead to loss of suspension. This prevents the residual limb from fully settling in, and thus structural rotation controls built into the socket will not be effective in limiting unwanted rotation.

An additional cause of this deviation would be weak hip musculature creating an inability to control both the prosthesis and the residual limb. Due to the hip being the most unstable link in the lower extremity chain at this stage in the gait cycle, dynamic muscular control of the femur is essential to prevent excessive uncontrolled rotation within the acetabulum, leading to observable lower extremity transverse rotation.

Excessive Toe-Out

Unilateral limb loss commonly leads to observable excessive toe-out on the intact limb. Although this can be due to a congenital gait pattern, it is disproportionately observed in the population with limb loss compared to the general population. The cause is a subconscious adaptation by the patient to compensate for their loss of balance and proprioception due to the pathology of limb loss. This compensation aids in maintaining center of gravity within their base of support. Interventions to treat this should focus on improving single limb balance on the prosthetic side and secondarily on the intact side. This is also the solution for bilateral lower extremity amputees who ambulate with this deviation, while having a proper prosthetic fit.

If excessive toe-out is observed bilaterally, it should be classified as a deviation, even though the patient may be moving symmetrically. If a prosthetic foot is externally rotated beyond the manufacturer's recommendations, the patient will not receive the energy return from that foot. Furthermore, persons with unilateral limb loss will experience abnormal torques on the intact knee, which will lead to poor gait efficiency and secondary complications [16].

Knee Buckling at Initial Contact to Loading Response

When observed on the prosthetic side, this would be from quadriceps weakness or prosthetic foot dysfunction in the transtibial population. For persons with transtibial limb loss, excessive prosthetic socket flexion or an overly firm heel bumper (or heel cushion) will result in this deviation. Prosthetic flexion can be simulated by an excessively dorsiflexed foot or by the socket being placed anterior over the foot.

During loading response, the knee joint is the most unstable point in the weight-bearing lower extremity chain. The implication of this fact for transfemoral prosthetic users is that the ground-reaction force can cause the prosthetic knee to buckle. Control of the prosthetic knee after heel strike relies on the intrinsic controls of the prosthetic knee along with the volitional concentric control of the hip extensor muscles. If symbiotically decreased activation of the gluteus maximus, and/or lack of intrinsic knee control cannot counteract the knee flexion moment, buckling will occur.

A hip flexion contracture or prosthetic alignment can also cause this deviation. When the soft tissue is shortened on the anterior hip, the gluteus maximus is functionally positioned at a mechanical disadvantage, while also promoting the ground-reaction force to sit excessively posterior to the knee. Prosthetic cause can include having the knee set too far anterior leading to a similar position of the ground-reaction force. Additionally, insufficiently designed socket flexion can lead to inhibited gluteus maximus activation. Prosthetic causes of early knee buckling may be overcome with patient compensation including increased ipsilateral hip extensor activation and/or forward trunk flexion to create a ground reaction force anterior to the knee.

Knee Extension/Hyperextension at Initial Contact to Loading Response

Knee flexion of less than the typical 15° to 18° is common for persons with lower limb amputations of all levels [11,17,18]. Hyperextension is typically associated with limb loss at the transtibial level. This can be propagated by weak quadriceps at initial contact as the ground-reaction briefly causes the knee to move into an extended position. Prosthetic extension can also cause this deviation, which includes excessive foot plantarflexion, lack of proper socket flexion, or a posterior shifted socket. In addition to alignment, prosthetic componentry including a worn-out or excessively soft heel bumper can lead to this deviation.

For the population with transfemoral limb loss, the observation of this gait deviation will typically be caused by prosthetic alignment. In some cases, this abnormality may be intentionally created by the prosthetist to prevent falling or to address a fear of falling, but should not be encouraged when a patient is using a prosthesis with a fluid-controlled knee.

Trendelenburg or Lateral Trunk Lean

Trendelenburg gait is classically due to gluteus medius weakness on the weight-bearing limb. Visualization of this deviation should appear as a slight lateral lean over the weight-bearing limb, and is due to a lack of ability to stabilize the pelvis during stance.

For persons with limb loss, this would typically occur on the prosthetic side, and pure Trendelenburg gait would be due to hip abductor dysfunction [9]. This lateral trunk lean can also be caused by a functionally or actually short prosthesis. If a patient is not wearing enough sock ply, the patient may bottom out in the socket and thus have a functionally shortened prosthesis. For persons with transfemoral amputations, pain in the groin area from medial socket brim impingement will also lead to lateral trunk lean as a pain avoidance compensation.

Knee Buckling in Midstance

Slight knee flexion from loading response to midstance of up to 18^0 is normal. This stance flexion is commonly observed in the general population. Stance flexion in theory acts as a shock absorber and can decrease impact and stress on proximal joints. Knee flexion to the point of buckling will occur if stance flexion cannot be controlled eccentrically by the quadriceps in patients with limb loss at a level distal to the knee joint. For patients with an amputation that requires a prosthetic knee, buckling can be caused by prosthetic dysfunction from either improper alignment (typically the knee is positioned too far anterior) or improper programming or setting of the knee joint stance control resistance. A patient with transfemoral limb loss with a hip flexion contracture is more prone to this gait deviation as the hip extensor muscles are in a position of mechanical disadvantage, as stated previously.

Excessive Knee Extension/Hyperextension in Midstance to Late Stance

Commonly described as genu recurvatum, this is typically an issue in the population with an intact knee joint. As the body moves over the limb, from mid to terminal stance, the ground-reaction force shifts anterior to the knee joint center. If this moment is overpowering, excessive knee extension will be observed. Prosthetic causes that lead to this deviation can stem from both prosthetic foot and socket alignment. An overly plantarflexed foot, toed-in foot, long toe lever, or hard dorsiflexion bumper (in an articulating foot), can all propagate genu recurvatum. Additionally, lack of appropriate socket flexion or posterior socket alignment can also lead to this deviation.

For the population with a transfemoral amputation, many prosthetic knees require full extension in late stance while loaded with the patient's body weight to trigger a shift in knee function from stance to swing mode. Hyperextension should be biomechanically impossible unless it is built into the alignment by the prosthetist.

Lack of Hip Extension in Terminal Stance

This is most common in patients with transfemoral amputations and hip flexion contractures. Shorter residual limbs correlate with increased incidence of hip flexion contractures. Asymmetry due to limited hip extension can be avoided with early interventions of positioning and stretching to prevent the contracture.

In terminal stance, the ground-reaction force moves posterior to the hip assisting in reaching an extended hip position. Consequently, this is a very stable position for a non-pathological hip. To take advantage of the stability of this position, it is common to have a hip prosthesis that is mounted (by design) on the anterior aspect of the socket for persons with hip disarticulation or hemipelvectomy amputations.

Drop-Off in Late Stance on the Prosthetic Side

This is typically a deviation that will be observed in persons with transtibial or more distal limb loss. Drop-off is due to an actual or functional shortened lever arm in the prosthetic foot. The lever arm can be actually shortened due to the foot being the wrong size, or can be artificially shortened by having an over-flexed socket, anterior shifted socket, dorsiflexed foot, or soft/broken dorsiflexion bumper (in an articulating foot). This can be correlated with full knee extension range of motion and good to excellent knee extensor strength in the residual limb. If the patient has a knee flexion contracture and/or weak quadriceps there is a possibility of knee buckling in late stance that may look similar to drop-off.

Decreased Push-Off in Terminal Stance to Preswing

Due to the replacement of the dynamic contractile tissue of the gastrocnemius–soleus complex across the ankle joint, with a simple keel, persons with limb loss have an inevitable loss of power at push-off [19]. The extreme of this deviation is easily observed as a lack of a crease in the forward third of the shoe on the prosthetic side. If this is observed, the patient is not maximizing the energy return from the prosthetic foot. A commonly expected compensation is increased hip extensor activation [19].

SWING PHASE DEVIATIONS

The ankle is the most unstable joint in the weight-bearing chain at terminal stance. Even though many prosthetic feet are non-articulating at the ankle creating inherent stability, proper dynamic alignment of the prosthesis is crucial to control the excessive forces acting on the ankle. The energy returned through the keel of the prosthetic foot relies on the position of the prosthetic foot in relation to the socket (or shank) and the ground to determine trajectory as the prosthetic limb transitions into swing.

Excessive Heel Rise During Early Swing

This can be considered "normal" for transtibial amputees [3], as this compensation assists in toe clearance as the lower extremity progresses towards midswing [12]. If heel rise is asymmetrical for the prosthetic side versus the intact side in a person with unilateral lower extremity limb loss, it should be very slight. In the transfemoral population, a slight increase can also be acceptable, and may vary based on the components [18], but in general excessive heel rise will create an unwanted lag in forward progression of the prosthetic limb.

Lack of Heel Rise During Early Swing

When this is typically seen in a person ambulating with a transfemoral prosthesis, the cause would be that the swing flexion resistance is too stiff and thus limiting heel rise. Knee flexion of less than 60° will also be common in a shuffling gait typical of someone with a step-to-gait pattern; a bad habit of forcefully thrusting the prosthesis forward with the hip flexors of the residual limb, or ambulating with a restrictive assistive device such as a standard walker.

Medial Whip

A classic gait deviation seen in persons with transfemoral limb loss is typically caused by malalignment of the prosthetic knee. During initial swing, the proximal segment of the thigh moves into slight abduction as visualized in the frontal plane. The key indicator of this deviation is that the knee points laterally and the heel of the prosthetic foot moves medially. The hip abduction is a compensation for the whip deviation, to prevent the person with amputation from kicking themselves with the prosthetic foot. The static lateral rotation in the knee alignment can be the result of incorrectly donning the prosthesis, or a loose socket that was rotated laterally.

If this deviation is seen in a transtibial patient it will typically be less pronounced, and may be from a poorly aligned prosthetic foot. Again, this can similarly be caused by an incorrectly donned or loose socket. A severe muscle length and/or muscle strength imbalance can be ruled out during the physical evaluation.

Lateral Whip

Lateral whip is the mirror image deviation of a medial whip. The thigh will remain underneath the pelvis in the frontal plane, the knee will point medially, and the heel of the prosthetic foot whips laterally. This deviation is caused by a medial rotation of the prosthetic knee, either permanently, or due to lateral socket rotation from a donning error, or loss of suspension.

Similarly to the causes for a medial whip in the transtibial population, causes would be prosthetic foot alignment, or severe muscle strength, and/or muscle length imbalance.

Dynamic alignment of a prosthetic limb is a key part of a prosthetist's evaluation of prosthetic limb fit. If at delivery, dynamic alignment is appropriate, it is likely that the patient needs further education in proper prosthetic limb donning or limb volume management using residual limb socks.

Circumduction

Thigh abduction is the key aspect of circumduction that differentiates this deviation from lateral whip. The knee, whether anatomical or prosthetic is extended, or very minimally flexed, throughout swing phase. The obvious cause of this would be a hip abduction contracture. In the absence of a hip abduction contracture, this would be a compensatory mechanism by the patient to avoid stubbing the prosthetic toe during swing due to a long prosthesis. The prosthesis may be functionally long due to loss of suspension, inappropriately applying too many residual limb socks, or an overly plantarflexed foot. In patients with transfemoral limb loss, an additional cause could be that swing phase resistance is not being triggered. This can be due to lack of weight-bearing into the prosthesis during stance, short step length on the intact side, or (in the newer microprocessor knees) the patient may have forgotten to charge the battery.

Vaulting

Vaulting can often accompany circumduction, as this is a sound-side compensation to clear the prosthetic foot during swing [6]. The key observation is plantarflexion during midstance on the intact limb while the prosthetic limb is moving through midswing. This occurs well before appropriate stance plantarflexion that would be visualized indicating push-off at terminal stance. As with circumduction, this deviation is often a compensatory mechanism to clear the prosthetic foot during swing phase due to a long or functionally long prosthesis. If this asymmetry is observed in a patient with a properly aligned and suspended prosthesis, the cause is likely due to a bad habit developed from a previous prosthesis that was too long.

Hip Hiking

Consequently, this deviation may accompany both vaulting and circumduction typically caused by a long prosthesis as well. The differentiation is that hip hiking is a lateral elevation of the pelvis on the prosthetic side during swing [11,17].

This is a necessary deviation for patients with a hip disarticulation or hemipelvectomy with a single-axis hip prosthesis. If the patient has prosthesis with a polycentric hip joint, the patient has the ability to achieve a more symmetrical gait pattern.

Long Step Length on the Prosthetic Side

Extremely common in persons with transfemoral limb loss [4,7,18,20,21], this asymmetrical gait pattern is characterized by a long step length on the prosthetic side and a shorter step length on the intact side. Accompanied by increased stance time on the sound limb in persons with unilateral limb loss [9,17,21], this deviation can be caused by decreased balance or proprioception on the prosthetic limb, fear of falling, or fear of weight acceptance by the prosthesis. Additional causes include lack of anterior pelvic rotation on the prosthetic side, a hip flexion contracture in the residual limb, or pain caused by impingement of the anterior brim of the socket. If a patient is a long-term prosthetic user, this deviation is sometimes caused by a bad habit from walking on a previous prosthetic knee that may have required full extension at heel strike to safely transition into stance phase.

PROXIMAL DEVIATIONS

Gait deviations that occur proximal to the residual limb can affect symmetry, efficiency, and overall gait fluidity [7]. Some of the following abnormalities can be targets of direct interventions, while others are secondary compensations to other dysfunctions such as decreased balance or pain. While the initial instinct is to focus observational gait analysis on the prosthetic limb and the lower extremities, it is equally vital to view the pelvis, spine, and upper extremities.

Lack of Anterior Pelvic Rotation on Prosthetic Side

This is extremely common in gait after limb loss, especially with more proximal amputations. This may be visualized as "kicking" the prosthesis forward using the hip flexors to initiate gait instead of anterior pelvic rotation. As the patient transitions from terminal stance into swing phase, initiation should be driven by the ipsilateral pelvis transitioning from its maximally posteriorly rotated position towards neutral. At midswing this progression should continue until the pelvis reaches maximal anterior rotation at terminal swing of approximately 5°. This is a rarely documented deviation during observational gait analysis, but is very common. If this occurs in early prosthetic use in the new amputee, this can develop into a long term bad habit. An impinging anterior brim on a transfemoral prosthetic socket, poor balance on the prosthetic limb, and/or fear of falling will also propagate this deviation.

Decreased Trunk Rotation

Moving up the chain to the lumbar and thoracic region, decreased trunk rotation is a potentially symmetrical deviation, which also makes it often overlooked. In quiet gait, the spine and pelvis will fluidly rotate in the transverse plane. If this is seen in patients who also present with decreased anterior pelvic rotation, it will be more asymmetric as the pelvis and thorax will rotate out of phase with each other [7]. Other gait deviations that lead to decreased trunk rotation include a wide base of support and decreased arm swing.

Excessive Lumbar Lordosis

Excessive lumbar lordosis is most common in patients with transfemoral limb loss. This is very commonly caused by a hip flexion contracture, and thus is often seen in patients with short residual limbs. Decreased stability produced by the transversus abdominis and multifidus muscles can also be an instigator of this deviation. Less common causes would be pain avoidance on a high, impinging anterior brim on a transfemoral socket, or exceptionally weak gluteus maximus. This can also be a secondary compensation to maintain upright posture when ambulating, while trying to maintain an anterior weight line on an unstable knee.

Arm Swing Deviations

As with other proximal deviations, this is also more common with patients with shorter residual limbs. Patients with limb loss may present with overall decreased arm swing, or upper limb guarding as commonly observed in gait of persons with decreased balance. Asymmetrical arm swing typically presents with the upper extremity guarding on the prosthetic side, with potentially excessive arm swing on the intact side.

CONCLUSION

As lower extremity limb loss technology continues to progress from carbon fiber energy storing and returning prosthetic feet and microprocessor-controlled knees into even more biomimetic technologies, the ability to achieve symmetry should be even more easily realized. Still, continued challenges will remain present in people with anatomical disadvantages towards achieving symmetry such as short residual limbs and loss of proprioception. Whether the individual is classified as complex, or is able to ambulate in a nearly balanced reciprocating manner, we must strive for perfect symmetry. The prosthetic limb and rehabilitation program that is prescribed must facilitate symmetrical mobility to preserve the proximal and contralateral joints from onset of pain and/or degeneration [6,22–25]. Delivering the most appropriate intervention is the process of observing an asymmetric or rigid segment during gait, diagnosing the cause through a thorough evaluation, and intervening to facilitate maximal symmetry.

REFERENCES

1. Hillman S, Donald S, Herman J, et al. Repeatability of a new observational gait score for unilateral lower limb amputees. *Gait Posture*. 2010;32(1): 39–45.
2. Skinner H, Effeney D. Gait analysis in amputees. *Am J Phys Med*. 1985; 64(2):82–89.

3. Perry J. *Gait Analysis: Normal and Pathological Function*. Thorofare, NJ: SLACK Incorporated; 1992.
4. Graham L, Datta D, Heller B, et al. A comparative study of conventional and energy-storing prosthetic feet in high-functioning transfemoral amputees. *Arch Phys Med Rehabil.* 2007;88(6):801–806.
5. Kaufman K, Frittoli S, Frigo C. Gait asymmetry of transfemoral amputees using mechanical and microprocessor-controlled prosthetic knees. *Clin Biomech.* 2012;27(5):460–465.
6. Sjodahl C, Jarnlo G, Soderberg B, et al. Kinematic and kinetic gait analysis in the sagittal plane of trans-femoral amputees before and after special gait re-education. *Prosthet Orthot Int.* 2002;26(2):101–112.
7. Goujon-Pillet H, Sapin E, Fode P, et al. Three-dimensional motions of trunk and pelvis during transfemoral amputee gait. *Arch Phys Med Rehabil.* 2008; 89(1):87–94.
8. Boonstra A, Schrama J, Fidler V, et al. The gait of unilateral transfemoral amputees. *Scand J Rehabil Med.* 1994;26(4):217–223.
9. Jaegers S, Arendzen J, de Jongh H. Prosthetic gait of unilateral transfemoral amputees: A kinematic study. *Arch Phys Med Rehabil.* 1995;76(8):736–743.
10. Lamoth C, Ainsworth E, Polomski W, et al. Variability and stability analysis of walking transfemoral amputees. *Med Eng Phys.* 2010;32(9):1009–1014.
11. Su P, Gard S, Lipschutz R, et al. Gait characteristics of persons with bilateral transtibial amputations. *J Rehabil Res Dev.* 2007;44(4):491–501.
12. Su P, Gard S, Lipschutz R, et al. Differences in gait characteristics between persons with bilateral transtibial amputations, due to peripheral vascular disease and trauma, and able-bodied ambulators. *Arch Phys Med Rehabil.* 2008, (7):1386–1394.
13. Hofstad C, Linde H, Limbeek J, et al. Prescription of prosthetic ankle-foot mechanisms after lower limb amputation. *Cochrane Database Syst Rev.* 2004;(1):1–42.
14. Zmitrewicz R, Neptune R, Walden J, et al. The effect of foot and ankle prosthetic components on braking and propulsive impulses during transtibial amputee gait. *Arch Phys Med Rehabil.* 2006;87(10):1334–1339.
15. *Pedorthic Reference Guide*. Washington DC: Pedorthic Footwear Association.
16. Beyaert C, Grumillier C, Martinet N. Compensatory mechanism involving the knee joint of the intact limb during gait in unilateral below-knee amputees. *Gait Posture.* 2008;28(2):278–284.
17. Sagawa Y, Turcot K, Armand S, et al. Biomechanics and physiological parameters during gait in lower-limb amputees: A systematic review. *Gait Posture.* 2011;33(4):511–526.
18. Segal A, Orendurff M, Klute G, et al. Kinematic and kinetic comparisons of transfemoral amputee gait using C-Leg and Mauch SNS prosthetic knees. *J Rehabil Res Dev.* 2006;43(7):857–870.
19. Yeung L, Leung A, Zhang M, et al. Long-distance walking effects on trans-tibial amputees compensatory gait patterns and implications on prosthetic designs and training. *Gait Posture.* 2012;35(2):328–333.
20. Maaref K, Martinet N, Grumillier C, et al. Kinematics in the terminal swing phase of unilateral transfemoral amputees: Microprocessor-controlled versus

swing-phase control prosthetic knees. *Arch Phys Med Rehabil.* 2010;91(6): 919–925.

21. Isakov E, Keren O, Benjuya N. Trans-tibial amputee gait: Time-distance parameters and EMG activity. *Prosthet Orthot Int.* 2000;24(3):216–220.
22. Kulkarni J, Gaine W, Buckley J, et al. Chronic low back pain in traumatic lower limb amputees. *Clin Rehabil.* 2005;19(1):81–86.
23. Taghipour H, Mohamamzad Y, Mafi A, et al. Quality of life among veterans with war-related unilateral lower extremity amputation: A long-term survey in a prosthesis center in Iran. *J Orthop Trauma.* 2009;23(7):525–530.
24. Struyf P, van Heugten C, Hitters M, et al. The prevalence of osteoarthritis of the intact hip and knee among traumatic leg amputees. *Arch Phys Med Rehabil.* 2009;90(3):440–446.
25. Norvell D, Czerniecki J, Reiber G, et al. The prevalence of knee pain and symptomatic knee osteoarthritis among veteran traumatic amputees and nonamputees. *Arch Phys Med Rehabil.* 2005;86(3):487–493.

21

Medical Management of the Residual Limb

Douglas Murphy

MEDICAL COMPLICATIONS OF AMPUTEES

Dermatologic Issues [1–4]

Folliculitis

Definition: Inflammation of the hair follicles of the skin. Hair follicles are damaged by friction or blockage of the ducts. Secondary infection can occur such as with staphylococcus or with a fungus.

History: The patient may complain of a rash, itching, pustules, and pimples near a hair follicle.

Examination: Shows areas of inflammation, crusting, or pustules around hair follicles.

Treatment: Hot moist compresses to promote drainage. Topical antibiotics such as mupirocin. Oral antibiotics such as dicloxacillin. Antifungal agents. Prevention occurs through reducing friction and keeping the area clean.

Epidermoid Cysts

Definition: Benign cyst caused by implantation of the epidermis into the dermis such as by trauma or surgery. They can become secondarily infected. They can be caused by a blocked pore. Alternative names include epidermal cyst, epidermal inclusion cyst, infundibular cyst, and keratin cyst. Often confused with sebaceous cyst.

History: The patient complains of a bump on the skin that may or may not be painful.

Examination: Can appear like pimples and pus may or may not be expressed from them. Often appear on skin that is relatively free of hair.

Treatment: Surgical excision. There is a cystic lesion with cornified epithelium and lamellated keratin. Hydrogen peroxide gel can be used to dry out the cyst.

Sebaceous Cysts

Definition: A closed sac under the skin filled with cheesy or oily material that most often arises from swollen hair follicles. Trauma can induce these to form. They are generally freely moveable, painless lumps beneath the skin. On occasion, they can become irritated and tender. May occasionally form an abscess.

History: Painless but sometimes tender lump beneath the skin.

Examination: May show the lump that may be red and slightly warm. A grayish white, cheesy foul smelling material may drain.

Treatment: Warm compresses. Injection of a steroid. Excision.

Eczema

This term is a broad one to describe many different types of dermatitis. The word comes from the Greek meaning to "boil over." All of the different types of eczema have a similar appearance. In the acute stage, there are small, fluid-filled vesicles arising from skin that is red and swollen. The vesicles break and cause a wet and oozing appearance. The fluid can then dry into a crust. For older lesions, it may be necessary to use a microscope to appreciate the vesicles. Eczema includes the following subtypes: allergic contact dermatitis, irritant dermatitis, fungal infections, scabies infestations, stasis dermatitis, dyshidrosis, nummular dermatitis, and seborrheic dermatitis. With respect to the amputee, several factors relate to the development of eczema. These would include fit issues with the prosthesis as well as edema and congestion in the residual limb.

Contact Dermatitis

Definition: This condition occurs when the skin becomes inflamed after contact with either a chemical irritant or an allergen. Thus the two subtypes of contact dermatitis are irritant dermatitis and allergic contact dermatitis. Contact with acids, soaps, detergents, solvents, or other chemicals can cause the former while the other is caused by substances to which the individual has developed an allergy. Allergens can include fragrances, nylon dyes, and components used in the creation of a prosthesis. The allergic reaction may appear from 24 to 48 hours after exposure. With some substances, the individual may initially tolerate exposure but after repeatedly coming into contact with the substance, a reaction develops. Other substances only cause a reaction with the additional exposure to sunlight.

History: The patient will report a rash that may include itching, redness, swelling, and tenderness. The patient may or may not be aware of a particular substance causing this reaction.

Examination: There is a rash that can include redness, swelling, tenderness, papules, vesicles, bullae, oozing, drainage, crusting, scaling and thickening of the skin.

Patch testing should include extra items that could be part of the prosthesis such as acrylic, polyester resin, and epoxy.

Treatment: Although in many cases the best option is to do nothing, in general the mainstay of treatment consists of removing the offending irritants or allergens through flushing with water and preventing further exposure once the agents are identified.

If the above measures are ineffective then steroid creams can be employed. These must be applied carefully because these creams can create problems of their own from overapplication. If topical corticosteroids are ineffective then oral medications can be used and one should be careful to taper these over 10–14 days. Alternative topical agents that might provide some resolution include tracrolimus ointment or pimecrolimus cream. Adjuvant treatments consist of wet dressings, antipruritic creams, and drying agents.

Superficial Bacterial and Fungal Infections of the Residual Limb

These occur relatively commonly due to the moist, warm environment as the residual limb lies in the socket of the prosthesis. Certain species of bacteria commonly populate this area; including staphylococcus epidermidis, staphylococcus aureus, and streptococcus. Inadequate hygiene and hot weather allow the bacteria and fungi to multiply. This bacterial overgrowth can result in superficial infections, rashes, folliculitis, and furuncles as well as more serious infections. Rashes and infections should be cultured and oral antibiotic agents chosen on the basis of the culture results. Topical antibacterial agents can be helpful if the condition is not too severe.

The environment of the skin in the prosthesis can also provide an ideal environment for the growth of dermatophytes and candida species. These superficial infections may respond to topical agents but a warm and moist status of the residual limb in the socket will work against topical agents. Systemic agents may be required.

Intertrigo

Definition: This is a rash that develops in areas of chafing on skin that is warm and moist such as the inner thighs and genitalia. A secondary infection from bacteria, fungi, or viruses can develop in areas where the skin is broken. Individuals who are prone to this condition are those who are overweight, diabetic, or those with artificial limbs. The latter tends to hold moisture. Friction between folds of skin in the distal stump can remove keratin. Superimposed infection or colonization can occur from candida species, fungi, bacteria, or viruses. Factors such as decreased immunity, incontinence, and immobilization can lead to this condition in the young and old.

History: Symptoms include itching, burning, and stinging in skin folds. Situations associated with increased heat, humidity, and strenuous activity can accelerate this phenomenon.

Examination: The skin may show erythema, maceration, weeping, crusting, pustules, and/or vesicles.

Treatment: Stump and socket hygiene should be emphasized. A barrier cream such as zinc oxide can be applied and the area can be left open to the air as often as feasible. The shrinker should not be worn at night for several days to help this condition to subside. Other options for topical agents are Greer's goo, antimycotic agents, and hydrocortisone creams.

Xerosis

Definition: Symptoms consist of dry, scaly skin that may be itchy. The condition is frequent in older individuals. Winter months may show a greater incidence.

Treatment: Patients should avoid drying out the skin through excessive cleaning with soaps, particularly through long baths. Applications of skin moisturizers should help.

Verrucous Hyperplasia

Poor distal fit in the prosthesis results in chronic tissue edema that has the appearance of warty papules. There is abnormal flow in venous and lymphatic systems. The histologic appearance is of pseudoepitheliomatous hyperplasia. In most instances, the condition is benign and reversible. Infrequently malignant transformation can occur. Mixed flora, bacterial contamination can occur from impaired immune responses due to the decreased blood flow. The best treatment consists of external compression and topical treatment of the bacterial overgrowth. Better distal fit of the residual limb in the prosthesis is imperative.

Acroangiodermatitis

Resulting from chronic pressure changes such as occurs with verrucous hyperplasia, this condition demonstrates vessel proliferation in the mid and upper dermis that is associated with red blood cell extravasation. Plaques and papules appear purplish and there is also skin that is edematous. One can use the same treatment strategy as for verrucous hyperplasia.

Hyperhidrosis

When the production of sweat exceeds the evaporation of dispersal of sweat, then accumulation occurs. Liners that impede the dispersal of fluid away from the stump can lead to this condition. Hyperhidrosis can contribute to other skin conditions such as the overgrowth of bacteria. This condition affects approximately 30% to 50% of amputees [8]. Studies on the use of botulinum toxin for hyperhidrosis have shown significant reductions [9].

Cleaning the Residual Limb

To help prevent dermatologic complications, the residual limb should be cleaned with soap and water at least daily. The preferred time for this cleaning is at night because the water will hydrate the skin and make it more susceptible to friction and shearing forces.

PAIN RELATED TO AMPUTATION

Residual Limb Pain [5–7]

The incidence of residual limb pain tends to decrease over time. The percentage of amputees having pain post surgery amount to 57% 8 days postoperatively, 22% at 6 months, and 10% at 2 years.

There are many possible causes of this pain. These would include infection, fractures, ischemia, tumor recurrence, surgical trauma, bony abnormality, entrapment of nerves within scar tissue, and neuroma.

Bony overgrowth can include growth of the distal bone such as in children, growth of the distal bone that results in irregular edges, and heterotopic ossification which is generally located at the site of bone transection. Heterotopic ossification can cause mechanical issues with socket wear and also be a source of pain. If heterotopic ossification causes problems with prosthetic wear or skin breakdown then socket modifications can help or resolve these issues. If they persist or worsen then surgery may be needed.

Tissue deformation of scar tissue that contains entrapped nerves may cause significant pain. Measures to control this pain could involve injections of steroid/lidocaine combinations as well as phenol. Oral medications might be helpful as well. Surgical options exist but these generally have not reliably produced favorable results.

Transected nerves at the site of amputation develop neuromas which consist of tangled, ball-like masses of nerve axons. Most neuromas are not painful and the incidence of painful neuromas ranges between 10% and 25%. Neuromas are among the most common causes of residual limb pain. Painful neuromas can be extremely sensitive to mechanical and chemical stimuli. Painfulness at a single point of palpation can strongly suggest the diagnosis. Ultrasound can confirm the presence of neuromas at times. An injection of lidocaine or some similar agent that eliminates the pain can help confirm the diagnosis. Treatment options can include physical modalities, medications, injection techniques, and surgery.

Physical modalities have not been able to provide substantial relief for neuroma-related pain. Examples of physical modalities include ultrasound, massage, transcutaneous electrical nerve stimulation (TENS), acupuncture, and adjustments of the socket.

Pharmacologic measures have utilized medications used for neuropathic pain. Typically these options can involve various types of tricyclic antidepressants, nonsteroidal anti-inflammatory choices, and drugs used for seizure control. Efficacy of these drugs has not been extensive.

Neurolysis can provide relief that lasts on average from three to five months. These injection and neurolytic techniques comprise at least the following: injection of phenol, cyroablation (freezing), and radio frequency ablation. As mentioned, lidocaine and steroid injections have also been used.

Surgical methods have been varied although not tremendously effective. Surgical techniques have included neuroma resection, sympathectomy, residual limb revision, and dorsal rhizotomy.

Pain Secondary to Prosthetic Issues [6]

Wearing the prosthesis can cause pain from multiple causes. Prosthetists generally fabricate sockets to focus more pressure on the pressure tolerant areas and relieve pressure on those anatomic areas that are intolerant of pressure. This strategy is often pursued even while at the same time pursuing total contact types of sockets. When excessive pressure occurs, the skin can develop signs of this situation such as calluses, blisters, breakdown, erythema, or even darkened areas.

In transfemoral sockets, if too much shrinkage occurs in the residual limb after the initial fitting and the wearer does not compensate sufficiently with extra socks, excessive pressure on the distal limb can occur and cause pain.

If suspension is inadequate so that pistoning of the residual limb occurs, pain during swing phase can make prosthetic use uncomfortable.

Poor fit of the transfemoral socket along the brim can cause impingement on bony structures such as the pubic rami or the groin area. Modifications of the socket are necessary to eliminate the pain.

Alignment problems can cause pain in many but related ways. If the foot is placed too far posteriorly in a transtibial prosthesis then excessive force from the quadriceps can cause anterior tibial pain as the patient attempts to compensate for ground reaction forces pushing the knee into flexion and potentially collapse. In a transfemoral socket placing the foot in an overly inset position medially puts greater stress on the lateral knee ligaments. The reverse can occur for a foot that is excessively inset laterally. Lateral and medial knee pain can result for these respective situations.

Such alignment issues do not have to result only in residual limb pain. Misalignment that causes the wearer to overly extend the lumbosacral spine can ultimately bring low back pain of varying severity and persistence to the wearer if the alignment issues are not corrected.

Phantom Limb Pain [4–7]

Definition: Phantom limb pain (PLP) is pain that is perceived in the absent body part after amputation. The incidence of phantom pain varies according to different studies. However, this incidence generally falls between 50% and 85% [5]. The relationship between preoperative pain and PLP as well as residual limb pain and PLP has seen variability in studies, some favoring an association and some that do not [5]. PLP can be associated with a diverse range of body parts such as the breast or bladder [5]. The pain can be perceived as throbbing, cramping, burning, or stabbing. The distal parts of the phantom limb may have a greater intensity to the pain. Factors that may worsen or provoke the pain could include certain positions, movements, psychological factors such as stress and sometimes the weather. The onset of PLP generally falls within the first 24 hours of the immediate post-operative period for about 50% of amputees and within the next week for 25%. However, occasionally PLP can develop weeks to decades later. It may lessen or even disappear with time but often persists.

Mechanism: The pathophysiology is generally separated into peripheral, spinal, and central causes. For some time neuromas have been considered as a causative factor. Neuromas can contribute but certainly are not the sole cause. Resection of neuromas may not eliminate PLP. The severed nerves from amputation can produce degeneration of C fibers in the dorsal horn. A fibers can branch into the lamina and then their stimulation might result in pain. Central mechanisms have not been fully clarified. Through the use of functional MRIs cortical remapping has been demonstrated in amputees and some patterns have an association with PLP. A neuromatrix theory [5] has been proposed to explain this phenomenon as a result of a complex interaction of the thalamus, limbic system, and cortex. This theory correlates sensory, cognitive, and affective inputs through a neural network with the brain. However, this model fails to explain all aspects of PLP such as why some people get it and some do not. Similar to the neuromatrix theory is a body schema model wherein the brain forms a schema of its parts that changes regularly as input varies.

Treatment: A large range of treatments for this condition are available. Few randomized controlled trials have been done, and fewer still treatments have shown effectiveness in these trials. Nonsteroidal anti-inflammatory drugs and acetaminophen are frequently used [10]. Treatments for neuropathic pain have been tried and used for PLP. These include both pharmacologic and nonpharmacologic treatments. Pharmacologic interventions have included antidepressants, antiepileptic drugs, local anesthetics, opioids, N-methyl-D-aspartate (NMDA) receptor antagonists, and transient receptor potential cation channel subfamily V member 1 (TRPV1) modulators. This is a receptor for pain and temperature.

Not all classes of antidepressants have proven effective. For example, the newer types such as fluoxetine, paroxetine, and sertraline do not appear to offer much benefit. However the tricyclic antidepressants such as amitriptyline and desipramine can provide benefit in these circumstances, although the evidence for their effectiveness is not particularly strong [5].

Examples of anticonvulsants that have some proven effectiveness are gabapentin, carbamazepine (brief stabbing pain [5]), and levetiracetam. Gabapentin has proven efficacy in some double blind, placebo controlled, randomized trials for neuropathic pain and in some cases PLP as well. There have been at least two studies; however, that did not show any effectiveness for gabapentin in PLP [5].

Lidocaine 5% patches can be useful for reducing neuropathic pain. One study showed the effectiveness of mexiletine in 18 of 31 people for providing some pain relief in those with PLP and there was a study supporting the use of clonidine and mexiletine in combination [5].

Ketamine is the primary NMDA receptor antagonist that has proven value in PLP. Thc oral agent in this class, memantine, has not shown benefit in some early studies but did in a more recent one as well as in some case reports [5].

Opioids have proven effectiveness in random controlled trials (RCTs) for neuropathic pain (for example, oxycodone, morphine, methadone, and levorphanol [10]). Long acting agents such as methadone or morphine sulfate controlled-release (MS Contin) should be used rather than those with shorter durations of action. Combining opioids with other agents such as tricyclic antidepressants can result in the ability to use lower doses [10]. Tramadol is a weak opioid and is also a serotonin–noradrenalin reuptake inhibitor [10]. It may offer an alternative with fewer tendencies for dependence and tolerance.

Local anesthetic blocks, topical capsaicin, and beta blockers have not been borne out in RCTs. Neither have surgical alternatives such as cordotomy and sympathectomy. Physical modalities such as TENS, acupuncture, vibration, hypnosis, and biofeedback have varied in their ability to affect this sort of pain in studies [5]. A recent case report suggests that pulsed radio frequency energy can help alleviate PLP [11].

One review [5] suggests that mirror therapy may be one of the most promising modalities or options for addressing PLP. A mirror is placed opposite the intact limb which is then moved and observed moving in the mirror in the location of the amputated side. Alternatively a virtual reality system can be used.

Interventional and injection techniques have results both favoring and disfavoring their use, and a wide range of treatments have been tried. Trigger point injections, sympathetic blocks, stump injections, peripheral nerve blocks, epidurals, subarachnoid blocks, and botulinum-toxin A injections have all been tried. Electrical stimulation modalities of the spinal cord including the dorsal columns as well as deep brain structures, particularly the medial and lateral thalamic structures have shown some effectiveness.

Psychotherapy, biofeedback, relaxation techniques, and hypnosis have provided some benefits. Temperature and visual feedback have been used as well as guided imagery and relaxation techniques [10].

REFERENCES

1. Wolff K, Goldsmith L, Katz SI, et al. *Fitzpatrick's Dermatology in General Medicine,* 7th ed., pp. 862–868.
2. Burns T, Breathnach S, Cox N, et al. *Rooks Textbook of Dermatology*, 8th ed. 2010;(2):28.7–28.9.
3. Meulenbelt HEJ, Geertzen JHB, Jonkman MF, et al. Skin Problems of the stump in lower extremity amputees. *Acta Derm Venereol.* 2011;91(2): 173–177.
4. Smith DG, Michael JW, Bowker JH. *Atlas of Amputations and Limb Deficiencies: Surgical, Prosthetic, and Rehabilitation Principles,* 3rd ed. American Academy of Orthopedic Surgeons; 2004.
5. Weeks SR, Anderson-Barnes VC, Tsao JW. Phantom limb pain theories and therapies. *Neurologist*. 2010;16(5):277–286.
6. Lenhart MK, ed in chief, Pasquina PF, Cooper RA, eds. *Textbooks of Military Medicine: Care of the Combat Amputee.* Office of the Surgeon General at TMM Publications; 2009, pp. 117–229.
7. Hill A. Phantom limb pain: A review of the literature on attributes and potential mechanisms. *J Pain and Symptom Manage.* 1999;17(2):125–142.
8. Meulenbelt H, Geertzen J, Dijkstra P, et al. Skin problems in lower limb amputees: An overview by case reports. *J Eur Acad Dermatol Venereol.* 2007;21:147–155. doi: 10.1111/j.1468-3083.2006.01936.x
9. Kern KU, Kohl M, Selfert U, et al. Effect of botulinum toxin B on residual limb sweating and pain. Is there a chance for indirect phantom pain reduction by improved prosthesis use? *Schmerz*. 2012;26(2):176–184.
10. Subedi B, Grossberg GT. Phantom limb pain: Mechanisms and treatment approaches. *Pain Res Treat*. 2011;2011:1–8. doi:10.1155/2011/864605
11. Garbellotti K. Pulsed radio frequency energy for the treatment of phantom limb pain. *Fed Pract.* 2012;23–25.

Index